D0893003

CLINICAL EFFECTIVENESS AND CLINICAL GOVERNANCE MADE EASY

Second edition

Ruth Chambers
and
Elizabeth Boath

Staffordshire
UNIVERSITY

RADCLIFFE MEDICAL PRESS

©2001 Ruth Chambers and Elizabeth Boath
Illustrations ©2001 Martin Davies

Radcliffe Medical Press Ltd
18 Marcham Road, Abingdon, Oxon OX14 1AA

First edition 1998

All rights reserved. No part of this publication may be reproduced, stored in a retrieval system or transmitted, in any form or by any means, electronic, mechanical, photocopying, recording or otherwise without the prior permission of the copyright owner.

British Library Cataloguing in Publication Data

A catalogue record for this book is available from the British Library.

ISBN 1 85775 443 3

Typeset by Advance Typesetting Ltd
Printed and bound by TJ International Ltd, Padstow, Cornwall

► CONTENTS

► ABOUT THE AUTHORS

Ruth Chambers has been a general practitioner for 20 years. She is currently Professor of Primary Care Development at the School of Health, Staffordshire University. Her interest in clinical effectiveness and clinical audit grew during her three-year spell as Chairman of Staffordshire Medical Audit Advisory Group until 1996.

Ruth has run several series of clinical effectiveness and clinical governance workshops, teaching a mix of primary and community care health professionals clinical effectiveness skills in easy steps and an understanding of clinical governance. The experiences of those workshops have informed this book.

Elizabeth Boath is the Head of the Centre for Health Policy and Practice at the School of Health, Staffordshire University. Her interest in clinical effectiveness grew from her time as a primary and community care research facilitator, during which she facilitated and taught on the series of clinical effectiveness workshops used to develop this book.

► ACKNOWLEDGEMENTS

The workshops and composition of this book were developed with a grant from the regional Evidence-supported Medicine Union (EMU) and funding from the Staffordshire and Shropshire Non-Medical Education Consortium, to improve evidence-based care in the West Midlands.

North Staffordshire Medical Audit Advisory Group were joint organisers of the clinical effectiveness workshop series and North Staffordshire Combined Healthcare NHS Trust was co-host of many of the clinical governance workshops.

The book is based upon the experiences from running two series of four workshops, *Clinical Effectiveness Made Easy*, for primary and community care practitioners and 20 workshops about *Clinical Governance*. We are grateful to the participants of the workshops for contributing so many ideas and being such an enthusiastic bunch of health professionals. Irene Fenton and David Rogers, medical librarians, provided the inspiration and clear advice about undertaking literature searches and other sources of evidence.

We are grateful to Nicky Macleod for her contribution about the meaning of cost-effectiveness, and Dr Gill Wakley who helped to devise and facilitate the clinical governance workshops.

Ruth Chambers
Elizabeth Boath
October 2000

'Many popular beliefs are either logically wrong or are not supported by evidence … There is no confusion more dangerous than the plausible.'

Normand C (1998) Ten popular health economic fallacies. *Public Health Medicine.* **20**(2): 129–32.

► INTRODUCTION

Clinical effectiveness and clinical governance are about knowing what you should be doing and being able to put that knowledge into practice

Overall aim of the programme

To increase awareness of, and skills in, the adoption of an evidence-based approach to the practice and delivery of healthcare.

Objectives of this book

This programme is for all health professionals to learn how to:

► ask the right question – it must be important to you and your colleagues
► look for the evidence and do a library search
► receive and incorporate constructive criticism from colleagues about their developing questions and search for evidence
► select the best evidence – what to do where none exists
► evaluate and interpret the evidence, such as read and extract information from a report
► apply the evidence as appropriate in a practice, unit or department

- ▶ act on the evidence to improve the practice of clinical effectiveness
- ▶ promote a culture of clinical governance.

▼

Do you need to update your style of practice?

Self-assessment of where you are now with clinical effectiveness and clinical governance

Before you start working through the clinical effectiveness and clinical governance programme, assess your baseline knowledge and attitudes. Please circle as many answers as apply, or fill in the information requested.

1 How confident do you feel that you are capable of practising clinical effectiveness to be able to:

ask a relevant question?	*Very*	*Somewhat*	*Not at all*
undertake a search of the literature?	*Very*	*Somewhat*	*Not at all*
find readily available evidence?	*Very*	*Somewhat*	*Not at all*
weigh up available evidence?	*Very*	*Somewhat*	*Not at all*
decide if changes in practice are warranted?	*Very*	*Somewhat*	*Not at all*
make changes in practice as appropriate?	*Very*	*Somewhat*	*Not at all*

2 Have you ever searched the literature yourself for an answer to a question?   *Yes / No*

   If '*Yes*':

   ▶ which database(s) have you used?

   Medline   Cochrane   Internet   Other (what?)

   ▶ where did you search the literature?

   Medical library   At work   At home   Other (where?)

   ▶ did you have any help in searching the literature?

   None   Medical librarian   Friend/family   Work colleague   Other (who?)

3 Have you ever asked someone else to search the literature for you?   *Yes / No*

   If '*Yes*':

   ▶ who did the search for you?

   ▶ why didn't you do the search yourself?

   Lack of time   Lack of skill   Lack of access   Other reason
   to databases

4 Can you complete the following list from your own knowledge, describing the features of different types or levels of evidence in decreasing order of robustness from very strong evidence to none at all?

Type	Features
I	Strong evidence from at least one systematic review of multiple, well-designed, randomised controlled trials
II	
III	
IV	
V	
VI	No evidence at all

5 If you have previously searched for the evidence to answer a question you had posed, what did you do with the result of your search? (Circle all that apply.)

▶ *Discussed it with colleagues at work*

▶ *Discussed it with friends or family*

▶ *Made change(s) to an aspect of work*

▶ *Decided against making any change(s) to any aspect of work*

▶ *Other outcome – what?*

6 To what extent is evidence-based healthcare central to your own practice? (Circle all that apply.)

▶ *I have no idea whether my everyday practice is evidence-based most of the time*

▶ *I assume that my everyday practice is evidence-based whenever possible, but I've no evidence for that assumption*

▶ *I ensure that my everyday practice is evidence-based by regularly comparing my practice against published standards of best practice and making appropriate changes*

7 How many of these principles of good practice in clinical governance do you generally include as part of your quality improvement work? (Circle all that apply.)

 ▶ *I actively promote or participate in multidisciplinary working*

 ▶ *I address national, local, organisational or professional priorities in my work*

 ▶ *I try to achieve partnership working, e.g. between agencies, between management/clinicians*

 ▶ *I incorporate input from patients in my work, (e.g. users, carers, the public), in training, planning, monitoring or delivery of healthcare*

 ▶ *I look for potential to achieve health gains in the way I organise my work*

 ▶ *My everyday work is based on evidence-based practice, policy or management*

 ▶ *I can demonstrate the standards of care or services that I or my team achieve.*

▼

Find out how to practise clinical effectiveness – don't shut your eyes to the changes going on around you.

What are clinical effectiveness and evidence-based healthcare?

Clinical effectiveness is 'the extent to which specific clinical interventions, when deployed in the field for a particular patient or population, do what they are intended to do – i.e. maintain and improve health and secure the greatest possible health gain from the available resources. To be reasonably certain that an intervention has produced health benefits, it needs to be shown to be capable of producing worthwhile benefit (efficacy and cost-effectiveness) and that it has produced that benefit in practice'.[1]

Evidence-based healthcare 'takes place when decisions that affect the care of patients are taken with due weight accorded to all valid, relevant information'.[2]

Evidence-based medicine is the 'conscientious, explicit, and judicious use of current best evidence in making decisions about the care of individual patients. The practice of evidence-based medicine means integrating individual clinical expertise with the best available external clinical evidence from systematic research'.[3]

A problem-solving approach based upon good evidence can also be applied to non-clinical decision making, such as most areas of management and resource allocation, as well as to clinical situations.

The three components of best possible clinical decision making[4,5] are *clinical expertise, patient preferences* and *clinical research evidence*. Clinical expertise and patient preferences may override the research evidence in some situations and for some patients. For example, patients may opt for less invasive treatment, or a sick patient may be too frail to undergo treatment with significant side-effects.

Clinical audit remains an important tool for determining whether actual performance compares with evidence-based standards and, if not, what changes are needed to improve performance. Clinical audit is 'the systematic and critical analysis of the quality of clinical care, including the procedures used for diagnosis, treatment and care, the associated use of resources and the resulting outcome and quality of life for the patient'.[1] In other words, clinical audit helps you to reach a standard of clinical work as near to best practice as possible.

The process of achieving evidence-based medicine can be divided into four sections:

1 the composition of a good question

2 a search of the literature to find the 'best' evidence available

3 an evaluation of what seems to be the most appropriate and relevant literature

4 the application of the evidence or findings.

What is the evidence for evidence-based healthcare?

There is growing evidence for the implementation of evidence-based healthcare.[6] Promoting Action on Clinical Effectiveness (PACE), a King's Fund programme, is developing evidence-based practice as a routine way of working for health services. An interim report[6] has described the successful outcomes when clinical effectiveness is linked to local needs and priorities so long as clinicians, managers, policy makers and patients are all involved in the process.

Practising in an evidence-based way:

▶ will promote your job satisfaction and feeling of being in control over your work

▶ can be used to justify maintaining or increasing budget allocations to particular areas of work

▶ will enhance your capability to do what's best for the patient.[7]

Why health professionals need information

Health professionals need to be well informed to be able to advise and inform patients appropriately. Patients who access the Internet and other electronic databases are starting to use that information to challenge clinicians' decisions about their care.

Clinicians will come under more pressure to respond to patients who have easy access to detailed information obtained from various sources, some of which will be inaccurate and misleading. The movement to patient empowerment has been generally welcomed, but may be threatening for clinicians who are insufficiently prepared to talk to well-informed patients, because they are unsure of their own knowledge base, time pressured, or do not understand how to assess what is the best evidence.

Clinicians will need to develop skills in finding and judging medical information, and communicating such information to patients appropriately. Health professionals may lay themselves open to complaints or legal procedures if they fail to adopt best practice through ignorance of the available evidence. Clinicians need good communication skills as well as reliable information when advising patients.

In the future, patients will be increasingly encouraged to seek out information from the Internet themselves. Health professionals can help patients by indicating which electronic sources are most likely to be appropriate and reliable.

Ultimately, reliable and accurate information, good communication skills and patient empowerment are all features of a good quality primary healthcare service and a positive culture of clinical governance. Health professionals and managers need good information when assessing the health needs of their patient populations, commissioning healthcare services, and striving to reduce inequalities, either between different sub-groups of their population, or between their patient populations and others elsewhere, or to reduce variations in performance between different practitioners and general practices.

▼

Quality of care may be compromised ...

▼

... without clinical effectiveness.

Are clinicians ready for evidence-based healthcare?

Recent surveys of general practitioners' perceptions of evidence-based medicine[7,8] found that GPs knew little about extracting information from journals, review publications and databases, and that few who were knowledgeable used these sources of information. Twenty per cent had access to bibliographic databases in their surgeries and 17% had access to the worldwide web.[7] But the majority of GPs welcomed evidence-based medicine and agreed that it improves patient care.[7] GPs have been found to be more aware of publications that summarise evidence,[9] such as *Bandolier* and *Effective Health Care Bulletins*, rather than electronic databases; fundholding GPs were more likely than non-fundholding GPs to have referred to these publications. The researchers[7] concluded that the way forward in encouraging primary care clinicians to adopt evidence-based healthcare lay in promoting and improving access to summaries of evidence, and encouraging those primary care clinicians who are skilled in accessing and interpreting evidence to develop local evidence-based guidelines and advice.

One study[8] concluded that what was needed was a culture whereby health professionals posed 'regular questions about the validity of patient care' and developed 'skills both in defining useful questions and finding the answers'.

When GPs were asked what training they wanted in evidence-based practice, just over half wanted training in the use of the Medline database.[8]

Adverse comments about evidence-based practice include fear of the imposition of too rigid a healthcare culture, the loss of an overriding duty to provide compassionate and sensitive care[10] and that wholesale evidence-based practice is unrealistic because it is not affordable.[11] Some people mistrust the research–evidence base component of evidence-based practice because of the unreliability of some of the published literature; study biases are not always sufficiently recognised or acknowledged and, in occasional cases, have been discredited by sensational scandals involving researchers falsifying data.[12]

A needs assessment of multidisciplinary clinical staff working in acute Trusts in the West Midlands[13] discovered significant unease about the conversion from a clinical audit to a clinical effectiveness culture, let alone the further evolution to a clinical governance culture. Several practical difficulties constraining the uptake of evidence-based healthcare were a recurring theme: poor access to information and electronic databases, lack of understanding about the definition and advantages of evidence-based practices, and the widespread need for staff training in critical appraisal skills.

The Get Research Into Practice (GRIP) project in the West Midlands[14] has described many ways to accelerate the adoption of evidence-based practice and associated skills. The Aggressive Research Intelligence Facility (ARIF),[15] which is a collaboration between public health, epidemiology, general practice and health service management centres, exists to advance the use of evidence in the provision of healthcare in the West Midlands region. ARIF's regular reports describe the reviews and appraisals of the evidence the unit has provided in response to questions posed mainly by purchasers. The answers can be duplicated when others request the same information.

Learning by portfolio

Portfolio-based learning has been promoted since the early 1990s as a style of education that allows individuals to progress at their own pace. People can adopt education relevant to their needs, and composing a portfolio allows plenty of opportunities for reflection. Portfolio-based learning is not an easy option[16] compared to relatively passive types of learning such as listening to lectures. It takes a great deal of effort to complete a successful portfolio built on your past experiences and to progress through the stages of gathering and processing new information, critical reflection, interpretation and application. But it is worth it. The satisfaction that comes from completing a portfolio is as much about being in control of your own education as is acquiring new knowledge, attitudes and/or skills.[17,18]

Another advantage of composing a portfolio is that on-the-job learning is relevant to your work and life, and this is likely to retain your interest. At the end of the project you will have discovered that you have further educational and developmental needs. You will then have to decide whether or not you have taken learning about this topic, as to how to practise clinical effectiveness, as far as your resources permit (time, cost and effort).

So, using a portfolio-based approach to acquire the basic ability to practise clinical effectiveness, you should aim in your work programme to:

▶ identify the learning task(s), e.g. what capability you need to be able to practise clinical effectiveness and clinical governance
▶ set learning goals, e.g. learn to frame a question; search for, interpret and apply the evidence
▶ identify ways of achieving your goals by, for example, working through this book, peer group discussion, visiting colleagues, undertaking a (supervised) library search, exploring the Internet, reading more widely, making changes at work. Use this information to compose your personal development plan
▶ identify learning resources, e.g. the books and electronic databases in the medical library, the Internet, books, journals, video tuition tapes, local courses, correspondence from hospital specialists
▶ monitor how well the learning is going, e.g. reflect on the development of your knowledge and skills, seek a colleague's view of your work. Work with others in your practice or at the trust, to feed your learning needs into the workplace development plan
▶ list your achievements, e.g. run through a cycle of clinical effectiveness
▶ use what you have learned, e.g. make change(s) at work as a result of obtaining evidence or new information as part of clinical governance.

Some people prefer to work alone, whilst others find that having a mentor to help build the portfolio is useful. A mentor can help to assess learning needs, develop a study plan, support and challenge the work done, identify further learning gaps, and generally help the person being mentored to stay on course. To some extent the way that this clinical effectiveness learning programme is set out obviates the need for a mentor, but if you think a mentor might facilitate your work, consider asking your local GP or Continuing Professional Development (CPD) tutor to act as a mentor; or maybe a colleague could work alongside you sharing the course too, as a 'co-mentor' or 'buddy'.[16]

▼

Clinical effectiveness requires real commitment.

Electronic databases

The Internet

The Internet is the largest computer network in the world to which almost any type of computer can link. Most academic institutions are connected to the Joint Academic Network (JANET) and its Internet service (JIPS); staff and students can then access the Internet free on campus, or can dial up from home via a modem for the cost of a local phone call. Once an NHS-wide network is established there is the potential for NHS staff to have similar access to the Internet.

Information can be extracted from the Internet or exchanged via the worldwide web (www) by electronic mail, telnet, newsgroups, network news, file transfer protocol and gopherspace (a system of interlinked menus which allows access to many Internet resources). The worldwide web is a system for providing access to a network of interlinked documents and information services across the Internet. Documents can be stored on the web as text, images, sound or video. The language that the web clients and servers use to communicate with each other is called 'hypertext transfer protocol' (http).

To use the worldwide web you need software called a *browser* (or *client*) to view www documents, such as *Netscape*. If you want to read more about searching the Internet, further details are given in the ABC of Medical Computing series.[19]

Various companies such as CompuServe and Microsoft Network offer online services. CompuServe provides access to shopping services, technical support, world news, and so on. CompuServe also links into the wider world of the Internet.

Medline

Medline is freely available on the Internet. It is free to doctors who are BMA members – join by completing a form on the BMA's website. Medline is available on CD-ROM or online via a PC (you will need a modem). It is produced by the National Library of Medicine in the United States.

Medline contains over 10 million citations dating from 1966 to the present, drawn from bibliographic citations and author abstracts from more than 4000 biomedical journals published in the United States and 70 other countries. Abstracts are available for about 70% of the entries. It covers the whole field of medicine, dentistry, veterinary medicine, medical psychology, nursing, the healthcare system, and the pre-clinical sciences. Coverage is worldwide, but most records are from English-language sources or have English abstracts. It is available free through HealthGate at http://www.healthgate.com/medline/adv-medline.shtml. Medline is also available on CD-ROM through Silver Platter and OVID, though beware as there are differences in search terms between the two.

Cochrane library

http://www.cochrane.co.uk. 'This [the Cochrane library] is the single best source of reliable evidence about the effects of healthcare'.[20] The Cochrane library includes:

▸ The Cochrane Database of Systematic Reviews (CDSR). These are structured, systematic reviews of controlled trials. Evidence is included or excluded according to explicit quality criteria. A meta-analysis is undertaken by combining data from different studies to increase the *power* of the findings.

▸ The Database of Abstract of Reviews of Effectiveness (DARE). This is a database of research reviews of the effectiveness of healthcare interventions and the management and organisation of health services. The reviews are critically appraised by reviewers at the NHS Centre for Reviews and Dissemination at the University of York.

▸ The Cochrane Controlled Trials Register (CCTR). This bibliography of controlled trials has been compiled by hand searches through the world's literature. The Register includes reports from conference proceedings.

▶ Only the Cochrane Database of Systematic Reviews (CDSR) is available on the Internet. The other titles from The Cochrane Library are currently available through Update Software's CD-ROM. Negotiations are currently underway to bring the other Cochrane Library titles to the Internet. So, hopefully, the full library will be available soon. Details of the Cochrane Library and CDSR are available online at http://www.update-software.com/cochrane/cochrane-frame.html.

EMBASE

The Excerpta Medica database (EMBASE) is one of the leading databases of biomedical literature that offers 13 comprehensive databases that are searched separately. These are: anaesthesiology; cardiology; drugs & pharmacology; gastroenterology; immunology & AIDS; nephrology; neurosciences; obstetrics & gynaecology; pathology; pediatrics; psychiatry; radiology & nuclear medicine; and rehabilitation. The references found in each database are indexed and abstracted from over 3500 biomedical journals beginning in 1988, but for drugs and pharmacology from 1990. It is updated monthly. Although over 40% of entries are drug related, EMBASE also covers areas such as health policy, drug and alcohol dependence, psychiatry, forensic science and pollution control. It is more up to date than Medline and offers worldwide coverage with a European focus.

Searching and browsing the titles of the references that your search finds is free. However, you need to pay to display the full reference (journal citation, author and abstract when available). EMBASE* is not a full text database, but you can order full text copies from this database for a fee. It is available at http://www.healthgate.com/embase/search-embase-pre.shtml.

CINAHL

The Cumulative Index to Nursing and Allied Health Literature (CINAHL) database, compiled by CINAHL Information Systems in the USA, is a comprehensive database of more than 1200 English language journals from 1982 to the present. Updated monthly, CINAHL covers all aspects of nursing and allied health disciplines, such as health education, occupational therapy, physical therapy, emergency services, and social services and healthcare. Selected journals are also indexed in the areas of consumer health, biomedicine, and health sciences librarianship. The database also provides access to healthcare books, nursing dissertations, selected conference proceedings, standards of professional practice, educational software and audio-visual materials in nursing. CINAHL has more than 7000 records with full text and 1200 records with images. Online abstracts are available for more than 800 of these journals. Approximately 70% of CINAHL headings also appear in Medline. CINAHL supplements these headings with 2000+ terms designed specifically for nursing and allied health. For more information, see the following website: http://www.cinahl.com. Email: support@cinahl.com.

Several studies have compared Medline and CINAHL. These revealed that while Medline assigns more index terms to each article, CINAHL uses index terms that are more focused on nursing and therapy topics.[21] Another study revealed that CINAHL was preferred by nursing students as it gave a higher number of relevant articles, while another study found that both databases were relevant for professions allied to medicine (PAMs).[22,23] The authors concluded that, in order to ensure that the search is comprehensive, *both* Medline and CINAHL should be used.

Subject-specific bibliographic databases[24,25]

Over 2 000 000 articles are published each year in over 20 000 medical and related journals. Thus, although electronic databases provide access to references from a large number of journals, no database provides access to all journals. So, if you search only one or two databases, you might miss a relevant article. In addition to searching the main databases, it is also worthwhile searching any specialist databases relevant to your area of interest. Some of these databases are outlined in alphabetical order below.

- **AgeLine** covers ageing, middle age and the elderly, and includes research on psychology, public policy, healthcare, business, gerontology and consumer issues. Searching and browsing titles only is free. AgeLine is available through HealthGate at: http://www.healthgate.com/res/index.shtml.
- **AIDSDRUGS** covers HIV and AIDS from 1980 to the present. It is free through HealthGate at: http://www.healthgate.com/res/index.shtml.
- **AIDSTRIALS** covers trials of HIV and AIDS from 1980 to the present. It is free through HealthGate at: http://www.healthgate.com/res/index.shtml.
- **AIDSLINE** covers references on HIV and AIDS from 1980. It is free through HealthGate at: http://www.healthgate.com/res/index.shtml.
- **AMED** (Allied and Alternative Medicine) is a unique database, only available on CD-ROM via OVID, that searches across the spectrum of complementary and alternative medicine. It covers reference articles from 400 journals, many of which are not indexed elsewhere, from 1985 to the present. For more information see http://minos.bl.uk/services/sris/amed.html.
- **ASSIA plus** (Applied Social Sciences Index and Abstracts) covers all major social sciences and related media including sociology, social policy, psychology and relevant aspects of anthropology, economics, medicine, law and politics. It features over 215 000 records from over 600 English language journals, covering 16 countries, including 25 of the 30 most cited sources. It covers the period since 1987 and is updated quarterly. It is produced by Bowker Saur and is available on CD-ROM. For more information see their

website: http://www.bowker-saur.co.uk/products/catalog/ a_and_i/assia_plus_c.htm.

▶ **Best Evidence** provides commentaries from abstracts that have been published in the *ACP Journal Club* and *Evidence Based Medicine* journals which provide detailed abstracts from published studies and reviews from 1991. It includes assessments of quality by clinical experts. It is updated annually and is simple to use, but provides incomplete coverage of the literature. It is available as a yearly subscription on CD-ROM from the BMJ Publishing Group (0207 387 4499) and at: http://hiru.hirunet.mcmaster.ca/acpjc.

▶ **BIOETHICSLINE** covers bio-ethical literature from 1973 onwards, including newspaper articles, books and court judgements. It is free through HealthGate at: http://www.healthgate.com/res/index.shtml.

▶ **CANCERLIT** covers the treatment of cancer and information on epidemiology, pathogenesis and immunology from 1976 to date. It is free through HealthGate at: http://www.healthgate.com/res/index.shtml.

▶ **EDINA BIOSIS** covers more than 6500 articles from more than 90 countries from 1985 to the present. It covers biological sciences and related subjects, including public health. It is updated every two weeks and over 500 000 articles are added annually. EDINA offers the UK tertiary education and research community networked access to a library of data, information and research resources. All EDINA services are available free of charge to members of UK tertiary education institutions for academic use. Institutional subscription and personal registration is required for most services. It is available at: http://edina.ed.ac.uk/about.html.

▶ **PsycINFO**® includes worldwide literature from 1967 to the present in the field of psychology and psychological aspects of related disciplines, including medicine, psychiatry, nursing, sociology, education, pharmacology, physiology, linguistics, anthropology, business and law. PsycINFO® is updated monthly and covers 1300 journals in 25 languages – over 45 000 references are added annually. Searching and browsing titles is free. It is available at: http://www.healthgate.com/res/index.shtml.

▸ **PsycLIT**® is the electronic version of *Psychological Abstracts* produced by the American Psychological Association. It contains 1 000 000+ records from over 45 countries in more than 30 languages covering psychology and related disciplines such as medicine, psychiatry, education, nursing, social science and pharmacology. PsycLIT indexes around 1300 international journals, plus dissertations, book chapters, books, technical reports and other documents from 1974 for journals and 1987 for books. It is available on CD-ROM and is updated quarterly.

▸ **SUMSearch** is a new method for searching the Internet for EBM information. It queries a variety of databases including Medline, the Merck Manual, the National Guideline Clearinghouse from the Agency for Health Care Policy and Research (AHCPR), PubMed and DARE. SUMSearch automatically corrects common abbreviations and common terms that are hard to search for on common databases. For example, it converts *DVT* to *deep vein thrombosis* and *heart failure* to *heart failure* or *ventricular failure* – small changes that greatly affect Medline. It is available free at: http://SUMsearch.uthscsa.edu.

Other information on the Internet [24,25]

▸ **Bath Information and Data Service (BIDS)**[19] at http://www.bids.ac.uk is a database designed to be used by non-expert searchers and includes several medically orientated databases such as Embase, Citation Indexes, and Inside Information, with a wide variety of medically related reference material.

▸ **Health on the Net** at http://www.hon.ch. The Health on the Net Foundation has developed a code of conduct for medical and health websites. This states that medical information should either be given by medically trained and qualified professionals or, if this is not possible, it should be indicated clearly that the information is given by non-medically qualified people. Websites complying with this code bear the Health on the Net logo. But the presence of a logo is not a guarantee of the quality of the information.

▶ The **Health Technology Assessment (HTA)** programme is a national programme of research established and funded by the Department of Health's Research Programme: http://www.hta.nhsweb.nhs.uk. Health Technology Assessments are peer reviewed, rapid systematic reviews, cost effectiveness analyses of health interventions and technologies which are produced by several groups.

▶ **Medical Matrix** at http://www.medmatrix.org. This database is published by Healthtel links, with around 4000 quality-assessed Internet sites of clinical medicine topics ranked for quality.

▶ Accessing databases of published research is easy. However, accessing information on research in progress is more difficult. The **National Research Register (NRR)** is a register of ongoing or recently completed research and development projects funded by, or of interest to, the NHS. It also contains details of reviews in progress collected by the NHS Centre for Reviews and Dissemination (CRD). The current release contains information on over 57 000 research projects, as well as entries from the Medical Research Council's Clinical Trials Register. The NRR is assembled and published by Update Software Ltd on behalf of the Department of Health in the United Kingdom. The complete NRR database is free on the Internet at http://www.doh.gov.uk/research/nrr.htm. It is also available on CD-ROM at local health research libraries. Further information is available from: The NRR Project Administrator, NHS Executive Headquarters, Research & Development Directorate, Room 5W34, Quarry House, Quarry Hill, Leeds, LS2 7UE.

▶ **PubMed** is the National Library of Medicine's search service that was developed in conjunction with publishers of biomedical literature as a search tool for accessing literature citations and linking to full-text journals at websites of participating publishers. It provides access to over 11 000 000 citations in Medline, PreMedline (updated daily and provides basic citation information and abstracts before the citation is indexed and added to Medline), HealthSTAR and other related databases, with links to participating online journals. Although PubMed is free, user registration, a subscription fee, or fee may be required to access the full text of articles in some journals. It is available at http://www.ncbi.nlm.nih.gov/PubMed/

▶ The **'NEW' TRIP** database is a one-stop search engine for evidence-based material on the Internet. It is an amalgamation of 26 databases of hyperlinks from 'evidence-based' sites around the world. There are currently over 10 000 links to evidence-based topics. It is available at http://www.tripdatabase.com/

Website for learning evidence-based medicine skills[26]

EBM at McMaster University at http://hiru.hirunet.mcmaster.ca/ebm/default.htm includes users' guides based on treatment and management of real cases.

Useful software

The Oxford Clinical Mentor[27] (OCM) is an electronic medical knowledge clinical support system developed by Oxford University Press with EMIS practice computer systems. It has information about more than 2000 diseases cross-referenced with about 25 000 commonly used medical terms. The programme comes up with a differential diagnosis for a set of symptoms, signs and test results, suggesting appropriate management plans which are a mix of evidence-based medicine and best practice. The information is regularly updated as new literature is published.

Electronic journals

All the titles listed below can be accessed free of charge. Some of the websites show the full contents of the journal, others do not carry the full text of all original articles.

▸ *British Medical Journal*
http://www.bmj.com
▸ *The Lancet*
http://www.thelancet.com

Full text journals are also available free of charge from the American Medical Association at http://pubs.ama-assn.org/ Journals available include:

▸ JAMA
http://jama.ama-assn.org/
▸ Archives of Dermatology
http://archderm.ama-assn.org/issues/current/toc.html
▸ Archives of Family Medicine
http://archfami.ama-assn.org/issues/current/toc.html
Archives of Facial Plastic Surgery
http://archfaci.ama-assn.org/issues/current/toc.html
▸ Archives of Internal Medicine
http://archinte.ama-assn.org/issues/current/toc.html
▸ Archives of Pediatrics & Adolescent Medicine
http://archpedi.ama-assn.org/issues/current/toc.html
▸ Archives of Surgery
http://archsurg.ama-assn.org/issues/current/toc.html
▸ Archives of Neurology
http://archneur.ama-assn.org/issues/current/toc.html
▸ Archives of Ophthalmology
http://archopht.ama-assn.org/issues/current/toc.html
Archives of Otolaryngology: Head & Neck Surgery
http://archotol.ama-assn.org/issues/current/toc.html
▸ Archives of General Psychiatry
http://archpsyc.ama-assn.org/issues/current/toc.html

'The greatest obstacle to discovering the truth is being convinced that you already know it.'

► STAGE 1

Asking the right question[28]

Although you may be burning to ask your question, when you actually try to set it down on paper, you may find that the exercise is more difficult than you think.

Questions have to be phrased in a very specific way to obtain meaningful responses in any context. This applies to asking other people what they think about a topic as much as for searching the literature for the best evidence.

The best clinical questions relate to queries arising from your own patients during the course of your work rather than being hypothetical questions. Relevant work-based questions should motivate you to seek the evidence and make change(s). Before you go to a lot of trouble to find answers or solutions to your questions, ask around at work and find out if anyone else is concerned about the same question or problem, already has the answer(s), or knows where to find them.

The question should be:

► simple
► specific
► realistic
► important
► capable of being answered
► agreed and owned by those who will be involved in any changes resulting
► implementable
► about a topic where change will be possible.

Think about how to construct your clinical question by considering:

▶ what the question is about. For example, is the question about an individual or group of patients? What are the patient characteristics you are interested in, such as age or gender? Is it a clinical dilemma or a resource problem?

▶ the setting. For example, is it specific to primary, secondary or community care, rural or urban locations?

▶ the type of intervention and whether it is being compared with current practice or another intervention. For example, are you interested in different treatments, causes, prognostic factors or risks, compared with current practice or no treatment?

▶ the outcome(s) of the clinical topic. For example, is an acceptable outcome to your question reduced numbers of cases of diseases, reduced patients' suffering, or increased quality of life?

You should focus and phrase your question to include whatever it is that you want to know about effects, efficiency, diagnosis or prognosis. You may decide to have a main question with several subsidiary questions.

Questions about cost-effectiveness

Cost-effectiveness is not synonymous with 'cheap'.

A cost-effective intervention is one which gives a better or equivalent benefit from the intervention in question for lower or equivalent cost, or where the relative improvement in outcome is higher than the relative difference in cost. In other words, being cost-effective means having the best outcomes for the least input. Using the term 'cost-effective' implies that you have considered potential alternatives.

An intervention must first be considered *clinically* effective to warrant investigation into its potential to be *cost*-effective. Evidence-based practice must incorporate clinical judgement. You have to interpret the evidence when it comes to applying

▼
Asking inappropriate questions.

it to individual patients, whether it be evidence about clinical effectiveness or cost-effectiveness.

If you want to ask a question about cost-effectiveness you should be sure to have confirmed clinical effectiveness first, and have gone on to ask a question about cost-effectiveness as the second stage in seeking the evidence.

A 'benefit' is what is gained from meeting a chosen need and a 'cost' is the benefit that would have been obtained from using the same resources in an alternative way. Opportunity costs are the costs of the benefits foregone in deploying resources in the chosen way.

A new or alternative treatment or intervention should be compared directly with the next best treatment or intervention.

An economic evaluation is a comparative analysis of two or more alternatives in terms of their costs and consequences.[29] There are four different types: cost-effectiveness, cost minimisation, cost–utility analysis and cost–benefit analysis. Cost-effectiveness analysis is used to compare the effectiveness of two interventions with the same treatment objectives. Cost minimisation compares the costs of alternative treatments which have identical health outcomes. Cost–utility analysis enables the effects of alternative interventions to be measured against a combination of life expectancy and quality of life, a common outcome measure being 'quality-adjusted life-years' (QALYs). A cost–benefit analysis compares the incremental costs and benefits of a programme.

Efficiency is sometimes confused with effectiveness. Being efficient means having obtained the most quality from the least expenditure, or the required level of quality for the least expenditure. To measure efficiency you need to make a judgement about the level of quality of the 'purchase' and be able to relate it to 'price'. 'Price' alone does not measure efficiency. Quality is the indicator used in combination with price to assess whether something is more efficient.

So, cost-effectiveness is a measure of efficiency and suggests that costs have been related to effectiveness.

> 'I have finally made up my mind but the decision was by no means unanimous.'

Framing questions: some examples

Now try these two examples of clinical situations and frame a specific question for each with which you might search the literature for evidence to answer the question.

Jot down notes under each heading and write the final question at the bottom of the page ready to do a trial literature search using the Medline database. Refine and limit the question to what would seem to be a relevant question for those working in primary care. Your question should be shaped by thinking out exactly why you are asking it and how you might apply the evidence in practice once you have obtained it.

Set a question to address problem 1

A general practice is taking stock of the preventive work it does and is reviewing whether to continue the range of work that different health professionals offer. The staff are wondering what the impact is of the range of health education about smoking that they offer their patients.

1 What is the question about – an individual patient, a group of people, a particular population, patient characteristics, a clinical dilemma, a resource problem?

2 What is the setting or context of the clinical topic/situation?

3 Is there an intervention and, if so, with what is it being compared?

4 What is/are the outcome(s) of the clinical topic?

5 What is the specific question you will ask?

6 Choose up to four key words, in priority order, that you think best represent the important components of your question and restrict it as far as possible to your field of enquiry.

Some example details follow.

Example details of question posed to address problem 1

Defining the question

The refined question should narrow down the limits of the enquiry by specifying as many of the following details as apply:

▸ What is the question about – the whole or a section of the practice population? What is meant by health education? Which staff are involved with the health education intervention? What is meant by 'smoking', etc.?
▸ What is the setting or context of the enquiry? The focus of your interest might be general practice, the community or primary care; or a particular type of clinic in the practice.
▸ Is there an intervention and, if so, with what is it being compared? What types of health education is the questioner interested in? Is there an alternative model to which health education is being compared?

▶ What is/are the outcome(s) of the health education intervention and what is meant by 'impact'? e.g. changes in attitudes, knowledge of, or quantity of, cigarettes smoked; reduction in disease severity or frequency.

▶ The specific question will have narrowed down the problem to one in which the practice staff are interested. For instance, if the staff in the practice were reviewing whether to continue the teenage lifestyles clinic, besides looking at attendance figures, patient preferences, and opportunity costs for staff, the practice team might want to know 'what is the evidence for the effectiveness of giving adolescents face-to-face education about the risks of cigarette smoking in nurse-run clinics?' A more general question might be 'what is the evidence for the effectiveness of a health professional advising a smoker to stop smoking?'

▶ Key words might be *health education, smoking, primary health-care, adolescents*, etc. depending on your question. You might have other key words.

Comments from participants' experiences at the live workshops on clinical effectiveness

Participants found that each small group composed entirely different questions as they had different foci of interests. Some found that their question did not contain the key words they selected after finalising their question, as they had not refined their ideas sufficiently. The result was that in some cases a later search on the chosen key words on Medline missed the point of the question.

Set a question to address problem 2

A mother asks a health professional about her child's eczema and whether it is worth going to all the bother of trying to minimise the amount of house dust lying around at home.

Have a go at completing parts of the question for problem 2:

1 What is the question about – an individual patient, a group of people, a particular population, patient characteristics, a clinical dilemma, a resource problem?

2 What is the setting or context of the clinical topic/situation?

3 Is there an intervention and, if so, with what is it being compared?

4 What is/are the outcome(s) of the clinical topic?

5 What is the specific question you will ask?

6 Choose up to four key words in priority order that you think best represent the important components of your question and restrict them as far as possible to your field of enquiry.

Some example details follow.

Example details of question posed to address problem 2

Defining the question

A refined question will narrow down the limits of the enquiry by specifying as many of the following details as apply:

▸ What is the question about – the child or the practice population as a whole? What is meant by house dust – or house dust mite? What is meant by eczema? Is there any other condition that it would be more important to search on, e.g. asthma?
▸ What is the setting or context of the enquiry? The focus of your interest might be general practice, the community or primary care, or a particular age of house.
▸ If there is an intervention, with what is it being compared – the method of eradication of house dust, or any other type of intervention such as other treatments for eczema?
▸ What is/are the outcome(s) of the health education intervention and what is meant by *minimise* – changes in symptoms, reduction in frequency of flare-ups, etc.?
▸ The specific question should narrow down the problem to one in which the mother and health professional are interested. For instance, to be able to apply her new knowledge, the mother will want to know the best method to use if the health professional advises that minimising house dust is effective. So you might ask 'what is the evidence for the effectiveness of measures to minimise the quantity of house dust mites on the severity of eczema?'
▸ Key words might be *allergy, dermatitis, eczema, mites, dust.* You might have other key words.

Examples of questions posed by the participants of the clinical effectiveness workshops

These are not given as examples that show particularly good or bad question formats, they are included here to show the range and variety of questions that individual participants in the workshops developed in conjunction with others in their practice or healthcare setting. These are the questions they used to search for the evidence, and when they found evidence, to interpret it and decide whether or not to put that evidence into practice.

- Is it cost-effective to screen all diabetics for microalbuminuria?
- Is the routine use of potassium-sparing diuretics in association with loop diuretics clinically justifiable?
- How effective is involving healthcare support workers (as opposed to qualified nursing staff) in continence reviews?
- Is there any evidence that a vegetarian diet reduces the incidence of bowel cancer?
- Do raised triglyceride levels have an adverse effect on diabetics? If so, what treatment is advised?
- Is an optimal outcome for patients with breast cancer treated by lumpectomy dependent on follow-up in a secondary care clinic?
- Are there any dangers in using mouthwashes?
- Is there a link between a history of potential tooth decay and the possibility of decay in children's teeth?
- Should maintenance doses of thyroxine be given in accordance with blood levels of thyroxine or the presence of patients' symptoms?
- Do practice registers of patients with coronary heart disease improve patient care?
- Has any work been published on integrated care pathways in leukaemia?
- What is the outcome of patients developing pneumonia who have had pneumonia vaccine over the past five years?
- Are head lice best treated by malathion or permethrin?

Clinical effectiveness is done best by involving the whole team.

Undertaking a library search

The search strategy: think, search and appraise

A search for the best evidence follows the sequence of 'think, search and appraise'. This search strategy comprises:

► thinking about and defining a good specific question in consultation with all the staff who are involved in the question and affected by possible change(s)
► searching for and finding the best level of evidence by looking critically at the relevant publications obtained
► appraising and interpreting the evidence as applied to your question in relation to your situation.

Clinical effectiveness encompasses the whole cycle:

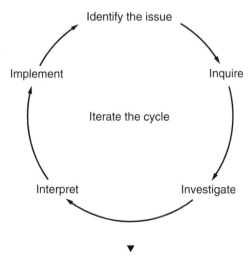

The clinical effectiveness cycle.

It is tempting for health professionals who are rushed for time and hot on the scent of evidence to a question to jump straight from an idea to carrying out a search, instead of working through the steps with the necessary rigour. Cutting corners wastes time in the long run if you ask the wrong question, answer a different question to the one you intended, or become distracted by lots of interesting but irrelevant literature.

How long you spend and to what lengths you go with a search will depend on its purpose. If you were commissioned to undertake a major systematic review, you would spend many months searching every relevant database, hand searching through papers and journals, hunting up conference proceedings, trying personal contacts, translating non-English language papers, and generally leaving no stone unturned in the pursuit of published and unpublished studies. But as you are probably a busy clinician who just wants to find the best evidence for answering a question in practice, you should strictly limit your search as your resources are limited. You will probably be better off spending your precious time doing several searches for different topics than doing one exhaustive search on a single subject. So stop your search as soon as you find a relevant systematic review of multiple, well-designed, randomised controlled trials in the Cochrane database. If there is no such systematic review in the Cochrane database move on to look for a review in the Database of Abstracts of Effectiveness Reviews (DARE). If no luck there try Medline, or Embase or other specialist databases until you obtain the best possible level of evidence that you can find.

If you have not undertaken a search of the literature before you would be well advised to book an individual session with your local medical librarian and to undertake a search in your postgraduate medical library if this is possible. You should be able to teach yourself from guidebooks, these notes, and trial and error, but a medical librarian is the person with the know-how about the best medical terms and phrases to try with your search. You as a health professional will know about the validity, context and relevance of search words and phrases as applied to your question. Together, you as a clinician and the medical librarian make a strong search team.

▼

Book up with a medical librarian to help you search.

Undertake a search

Before you start *write down* the key words you want to use and prioritise their order of importance. How many key words you enter as the first stage depends on how wide you expect your field of enquiry to be. If you key in *asthma* you would expect to identify thousands more references to published papers than if you keyed in the name of a rare condition. So if you are searching within a broad topic area such as *asthma* you should prepare more potential words to narrow the field of your search for the few most relevant papers that will supply evidence to answer your original question. Refine your question prior to your search so that it is very focused and make sure that the key words are the most pertinent you can manage. Then you will spend less time on your search and have more chance of finding the most appropriate published evidence. So if you want to know more in the subject area of *asthma*, build your question carefully. Aim specifically at the purpose of the question and include the setting, the population under question, the intervention, the outcome and any other important details.

In order to help in the search for evidence, a number of redefined search strategies have been published. These are a tailored set of instructions for locating randomised controlled trials (RCTs), systematic reviews, meta-analyses etc. Systematic reviews on Medline and CINAHL can be found at http://www.york.ac.uk/inst/crd/search.htm. Other search strategies including those for RCTs are available at http://www.ncbi.nlm.nih.gov/PubMed/clinical.html.

Using the Cochrane database

Enter your most important key words first – perhaps two words, as there are relatively few publications on the Cochrane database compared to other databases. Look at the different levels of evidence from the systematic reviews on the Cochrane Database of Systematic Reviews (CDSR) to controlled trials on the Cochrane Controlled Trials Register (CCTR) to the abstracts on the Database of Abstracts of Reviews of Effectiveness (DARE). The hierarchy of evidence is explained further in the next section.

It is likely that you will obtain only a small number of references to relevant-sounding systematic reviews because, as mentioned above, the Cochrane has relatively few publications on its databases in comparison to others. It is more likely that you will not find a relevant systematic review, but will identify many references to controlled trials. You should then modify your search further by entering the first two key words again plus a third key word that was your next choice in priority order in your original list of key words constructed prior to beginning your search. If this has not refined your search enough, repeat the exercise, adding a fourth key word. When you have narrowed your search sufficiently, print off the abstracts of the papers you have identified and obtain copies of the original articles as appropriate so that you can critically appraise them yourself.

Do not assume that the contents of any paper published in a journal are valid, reliable or accurate, however reputable the journal. Mistakes may have been overlooked, studies reported might not be relevant to your own situation, or the results may not be generalisable to your question.

If your search on the Cochrane database has been unsuccessful, move on to another database which has many more references to medical publications, such as Medline.

Using the Medline database

Because Medline has a phenomenal number of references you will have to develop a very strict search strategy to narrow down your focus of enquiry. To operate a search on Medline, you can use the key words that occur in its thesaurus of medical terms, the medical subject heading list (MeSH). There are over 17 500 MeSH terms arranged as a tree structure with broad subject areas branching off and sub-dividing into narrower subject terms. If you key in a word which is not a MeSH term, Medline will give you a choice of terms with close meanings. For instance if you key in 'primary care', which is not a key word in MeSH, Medline offers you 'primary healthcare', amongst others; if you key in 'cigarettes', which is not a key word in MeSH, Medline will give you 'smoking', 'smoking cessation' or 'cannabis smoking' as alternative words or phrases.

You can trace published literature on Medline by either searching for your own key word(s) in the title, abstract, author's name, or body of any articles or papers, or by searching for articles containing selected words from the MeSH list.

Entering one key word will often yield thousands of references to published articles. So, you can do a more selective search by combining key words using the instructions 'and' and 'or' (these are called Boolean operators). To narrow the search further you can restrict the numbers of years of literature searched, the language the paper is written in, the papers in the journals of the abridged *Index Medicus*, and specify 'human' as opposed to 'animal' research.

In a medical library, all you will need to do to access Medline or the Cochrane databases is to click on the icons on your screen, signposting you to the relevant databases. You may use Ovid software or another standard communications programme to access the Medline service.

There are two publications which give easy-to-follow practical details of undertaking a Medline search[30,31] which you could consult if you are unfamiliar with Medline searching and want to read more about the process before having a go for yourself.

Hints for the use of Medline (adapted from Ovid Technologies software) are:

▸ click on a **Subject Heading** to view its tree of key words or terms

▸ select the **Explode** box to retrieve references using your selected key word and all the more specific terms stemming from it

▸ select the **Focus** box to limit your search to those documents in which your key word (subject heading) is considered to be the main point of the article

▸ if the topic of your search does not map to a desirable subject heading, click on the box **Search as Keyword**.

You will learn most by having a go. You really cannot do anything wrong that you are not able to put right by retracing your steps. There are help boxes and icons throughout the database forms.

The hierarchy of evidence

The table below shows the generally agreed strengths of evidence ranging from level I, which is the most robust evidence, to level V based on the opinions of experts in the field.[28] But there may not be any evidence in the literature for answering the question(s) you are posing.

Type	Evidence
I	Strong evidence from at least one systematic review of multiple, well-designed, randomised controlled trials
II	Strong evidence from at least one properly designed, randomised controlled trial of appropriate size
III	Evidence from well-designed trials without randomisation, single group pre–post, cohort, time series or matched case–control studies
IV	Evidence from well-designed non-experimental studies from more than one centre or research group
V	Opinions of respected authorities, based on clinical evidence, descriptive studies or reports of expert committees

The most valid types of research for extracting evidence about clinical effectiveness are randomised controlled trials, followed by controlled trials, then trials and, less reliably, observational studies. A systematic review of several randomised controlled studies or all known studies is better than a review of some studies, which in turn is better than a report of a case study. You should start to search for the best evidence and, if you do not find it, work down the hierarchy.

If there is no reliable evidence to be found after searching the Cochrane, Medline and other relevant databases, you should then move on to look for any expert consensus agreements by multidisciplinary groups.

Be realistic – try and find one or a few key reviews rather than get bogged down in a plethora of papers. Clinical effectiveness is a tool for keeping up to date with your clinical practice, retaining your professional interest and enhancing your effectiveness – spending too much time pursuing it may be counterproductive.

> 'Most of my problems either have no answer or else the answer is worse than the problem.'

Examples

Example of literature search using problem 1 described previously

Question: What is the evidence for the effectiveness of a health professional advising a smoker to stop smoking?

Key words: *health education, smoking, primary healthcare, family practice*

Selected Medline database <1997 to April 2000>

The search used the MeSH words *health education, smoking, primary healthcare, family practice* fed in one at a time to build up the search.

Set	Search	Results
1	explode *health education*/	8454
2	explode *smoking*/	7804
3	(combine) 1 and 2	246
4	limit 3 to English language	212
5	explode *primary healthcare*/	4878
6	*family practice*/	5543
7	(combine) 5 or 6	9864
8	(combine) 4 and 7	11

Use IT to ask a question and search for the evidence systematically.

The searcher has limited the search to recent papers published from 1997 onwards. Sets 1 and 2 show how many papers were held by Medline where *health education* and *smoking* were listed on the database. Someone who does not know the subject field very well may use the command 'explode' to access all possible articles on the database, to avoid restricting the search to a subsection of the Medline database 'tree'. Using the 'explode' function avoids relying on the MeSH indexer, with whose categorisation you may not agree.

Set 3 combines *health education* and *smoking* to find those 246 papers where both these key words appear. Set 4 confines the references obtained in the search to those 212 publications written in English. There are still too many abstracts to browse through to find relevant papers. So, to modify the search further and focus on the most relevant papers, the searcher added *primary healthcare* in set 5 and *family practice* in set 6 to specify the setting in which *health education* and *smoking* was of interest. The search word *primary healthcare* has several branches and that is why the searcher has 'exploded' it in set 5 so that none of the branches are missed; but *family practice* is at the end of a branch and has therefore not been 'exploded'. The reason that both *primary healthcare* and *family practice* were included was that papers from inside and outside the UK were of interest and many countries such as the USA might be more likely to use the term *family practice* in place of *primary healthcare*. Keying in *primary healthcare* or *family practice* found 9864 papers, and many publications would have been missed if only one of these terms had been used.

By combining sets 4 and 7 (that is, looking for papers in English that have key words *health education* and *smoking* and *primary healthcare* or *family practice*), references were found to 11 papers. It is realistic to scroll through this number of abstracts to look for relevant publications. So the search could stop here if enough relevant material has been identified.

A further modification by exploding and adding *smoking cessation* would not have found any more references as *smoking cessation* is a branch of *smoking*.

A search may be narrowed further by introducing the word 'not' and by linking adjacent words that might equally well stand alone.[30]

An experienced medical librarian is an invaluable guide for a novice searcher. Besides knowing alternative terms such as *family practice* and *primary healthcare* as already described, the librarian will be aware of what words may be spelt differently by researchers in different countries, likely categories for your subject areas, and which databases are most appropriate for the topic of your search.

Example of literature search using problem 2 described previously

Question: What is the evidence for the effectiveness of measures to minimise the quantity of house dust mites on the severity of eczema?

Key words: *allergy, dermatitis, eczema, mites, dust*

Cochrane database: 2000, Issue 1

If the advanced search option is tried, using one of the key words *eczema* or *dermatitis* and, in addition, *mite** (using the * after mite means that if mite is only a part of the word included in the database the reference will still appear), 339 references are identified for *mite**, 1111 with the key word *dermatitis*, and 491 for *eczema*. Using a combination of *dermatitis* or *eczema*, 1374 'hits' are scored; adding *mite** at this point gains 32 'hits' – one systematic review (CDSR), two protocols, no abstracts of reviews (DARE), and 27 references to controlled trials (CCTR), of which three seem appropriate:

▸ Tan BB, Weald D, Strickland I, Friedmann PS (1996) Double-blind controlled trial of effect of house-dust mite allergen avoidance on atopic dermatitis. *Lancet.* **347**: 15–18.

► Friedmann PS, Tan BB (1998) Mite elimination – clinical effect on eczema. *Allergy.* **53**(48 Suppl): 97–100.
► Hide DW, Matthews S, Matthews L *et al.* (1994) Effect of allergen avoidance in infancy on allergic manifestations at age two years. *J Allergy Clin Immunol.* **93**: 842–6.

A 'belt and braces' technique makes sure you do not miss anything and you might key in '*dust.tx*' instead. This identifies any article on the database where *dust* is a textword (*tx*) that appears in the abstract. This reduces your reliance on the Cochrane indexer and minimises your chances of missing any paper relating to *house dust* that an indexer has categorised differently to the way in which you would have expected.

Medline database

Selected Medline database <1997 to April 2000>

Set	Search	Results
1	explode *eczema/*	293
2	explode *dermatitis/*	4878
3	(alternative)1 or 2	4878
4	explode *mites/*	829
5	(combine) 3 and 4	65
6	*dust/*	976
7	*dust.tw*	1626
8	6 or 7	1857
9	5 and 8	37
10	limit 9 to English language	32

Exploding the key words *dermatitis* and *eczema* in sets 1 and 2 and then combining them in set 3 ensures that all papers are identified where either the word *eczema* or *dermatitis* is used. Take care about keying in 'and' and 'or'. Keying in '1 and 2' in set 3 would have meant that identified articles must contain both of those words, which was obviously not the intention of the search.

Modifying the search in set 5 by adding *mites* found 65 papers. Adding *dust* modified the search further so that by set 10 there were 32 papers. The searcher did not explode *dust* on this occasion, because *dust* is one of the MeSH words in the Medline database, with many irrelevant branches such as *cosmic dust* which, if followed, would identify similarly irrelevant papers. The searcher had already noted that *dust* on Medline included *house dust* as a branch. To reduce the chances of missing any relevant papers, the searcher used the textword abbreviated as *dust.tw* to identify an extra 650 papers (1626–976) where *dust* appeared anywhere in the text on the database but had not been classified as a MeSH word by the Medline cataloguer.

Browsing through the 32 abstracts on the screen found five that looked interesting. One of these seemed very relevant to the question:

► Friedmann PS, Tan BB (1998) Mite elimination – clinical effect on eczema. *Allergy*. **53**(48 Suppl): 97–100.

This is an example of a search strategy that has been designed not to miss any papers by starting out to look as widely as possible for references and then gradually narrowing down the search. If the searcher had keyed in the instruction to *focus* on '*dust*', this might have been exclusive.

It is a good idea to print out the results of your search before you leave the screen, making concurrent notes on the paper print-out to remind you of the stages of your search, otherwise it will be a meaningless jumble at the end.

Example of search using one of the workshop participant's questions

Question: Is it cost-effective to screen all diabetics for micro-albuminuria?

Key words: *microalbuminuria, diabetes mellitus, screening, cost-effectiveness*

Cochrane database: 2000, Issue 1

Keying in the umbrella term *diabet* * ensured that papers with the words *diabetic, diabetes, different types of diabetes* were all included.

Similarly the key word *microalbumin* * ensured that words with slightly different endings were all included. Browsing through the MeSH headings for *diabet* * in the Cochrane database reveals many specific types of diabetes in the thesaurus. Keying in *diabet* * found 8764 references, whilst *diabetes* found 6707 references.

There was a total of 284 'hits' from searching on *microalbumin* * and *diabet* * in the Cochrane database. Six were 'hits' on the Cochrane Database of Systematic Reviews (CDSR), of which four were complete reviews and two were protocols of reviews. There were references to 270 controlled trials in the Cochrane Controlled Trials Register (CCTR) and one 'hit' on the Database of Abstracts of Reviews of Effectiveness (DARE).

Modifying the search by adding the term *screen* * reduced the number of controlled trials to 14 with one protocol featured in the CDSR and one complete review.

Under 'other sources of information', the NHS Economic Evaluation Database (NHS EED) produced five 'hits' of which the following paper was particularly relevant:

▸ Le Floch JP, Charles MA, Philippon C, Perlemuter L (1994) Cost-effectiveness of screening for microalbuminuria using immunochemical dipstick tests or laboratory assays in diabetic patients. *Diabetic Medicine*. **11**: 349–56.

Medline search: 1997 to April 2000

The word *microalbuminuria* did not exist in the MeSH index – *albuminuria* was the nearest match. Keying in *diabetes* gave a selection of search words in the MeSH index under the umbrella term *diabetes* of *diabetes insulin dependent, diabetic neuropathies, hypertension, diabetes mellitus, cardiovascular diseases, risk factors, blood pressure, diabetic angiopathies, urinary tract infections;* the searcher chose to select *diabetes mellitus*.

Keying in the word *screening* gave a choice of *mass screening, substance-related disorders, breast screening, cerebral aneurysm, diabetic retinopathy, colonoscopy, chlamydia trachomatis, neisseria gonorrhoea, sensitivity and specificity, colorectal neoplasm, diagnostic services* and *preventive health services.*

The table below describes the results of the search on Medline for evidence to answer the same question:

Set	Search	Results
1	*albuminuria/*	955
2	explode *diabetes mellitus/*	18 682
3	1 and 2	630
4	explode *mass screening/*	9528
5	*screen$.tw*	30 012
6	explode *preventive health services/*	18 758
7	4 or 5 or 6	43 191
8	3 and 7	57
9	limit 8 to English language	51

The search might be narrowed further by adding another modification, 'aim', which stands for 'Abridged *Index Medicus*', but these are mainly American journals and by doing this, you might miss UK-based publications.

This search demonstrates a strategy nicknamed 'building a hedge'. This will capture any references categorised under *mass screening, preventive health services* or *screening*, to cover all categories that the indexer might have selected according to MeSH headings. The term *screen$* is the equivalent way of displaying terms on Medline as *screen** is on the Cochrane database, to cover all key words starting with *screen*.

The great care necessary to avoid missing relevant publications is illustrated by the following example of a paper not being categorised under *screening* in the MeSH categories in Medline despite it having this word in its title:

▶ Kiberd BA, Jindal KK (1995) Screening to prevent renal failure in insulin-dependent diabetic patients: an economic evaluation. *BMJ.* **311**: 1595–9.

The paper was identified by the Cochrane Library search. However, it was actually inconclusive because the study population was limited to insulin-dependent diabetes and so it did not answer the question. But the only way it would be identified in a Medline search would be by the searcher setting up the instruction to search for all abstracts containing the key word *screen$.tw.*

Coincidentally, the medical librarian helping with this search remembered seeing a relevant paper in the local area's postgraduate journal:

▶ Davies S (1997) Microalbuminuria. *Midlands Medicine*. **20**: 67–9.

This was a very helpful paper which was not held on either of the Cochrane or Medline databases searched, being part of the 'grey' literature. It was consistent with level V in the hierarchy of evidence, describing the opinion of a local well-informed expert who stated that 'microalbuminuria has been identified as the strongest predictor of diabetic nephropathy, with 80–90% of affected patients going on to develop this problem' and recommended annual screening of diabetics aged 12–70 years for microalbuminuria. This article cited four other relevant references, all of which were published before 1997, and had therefore been missed in this Medline search which had been limited to published papers from 1997 onwards.

Another useful way of limiting a search is to see if your searching facilities permit you to confine your search to 'local holdings' of literature so that you can easily refer to original papers once you have identified the references from your computerised search.

As a result of the evidence gained from the search, the workshop participant who posed this question instituted routine testing of diabetics for microalbuminuria in the practices' protocols.

▼
Information is power!

Example of search using a second workshop participant's question

Question: Is an optimal outcome for patients with breast cancer treated by lumpectomy dependent on follow-up in a secondary care clinic?

Key words: *breast cancer, lumpectomy, follow-up*

Cochrane database: 2000, Issue 1

The MeSH term *Breast Neoplasms* identified 2613 references. As the MeSH term might not identify all controlled trials, '*Breast Neoplasm**' was searched as a textword using the 'Advanced Search' option and produced 3143 references. Putting a phrase in inverted commas like this ensures that it is searched as a phrase. In order to be comprehensive, '*breast cancer*' was added and produced 4416 references. Combining the three searches above using the term 'or' produced 5087 references (set 1).

The MeSH term *mastectomy-segmental* was added and produced 119 references. Adding *lumpectomy* as a textword identified 115 references and combining these above using the term 'or' gave 195 (set 2). The MeSH term *follow-up* gave the subcategory *follow-up-studies* which, when chosen, gave 12 369 references and textword *follow-up* produced 623. Combining these above using the term 'or' gave 12 845 references (set 3). Finally, combining sets 1, 2 and 3 using the term 'and' gave 35 references.

This revealed 33 'hits' on the CCTR, one review on DARE and one hit on the NHS Economic Evaluation Database (NHS EED). As little appropriate information was obtained from the search and the abstracts obtained did not appear to address the question, the searcher moved on to search Medline.

It is important not to narrow your search too much at the beginning to restrict yourself unnecessarily or risk missing papers that the indexer of the database categorised in a different way from that which you would have expected.

Medline database

Keying in *breast cancer* gave a choice of *breast neoplasm/mass screening/mammography/adenocarcinoma/proteins/antineoplastic agents, hormonal/case-control studies/age factors/antineoplastic agents, combined/tamoxifen. Lumpectomy* was not a word recognised in Medline; the options given were *mastectomy* or *mastectomy, segmental*, and the latter was chosen.

The search word *follow-up* resulted in a choice of *follow-up studies/coronary disease/laryngeal nerves/cornea/depressive disorder/ aged 80 or over/aging/factor viii/treatment outcome/myopia*, from which *follow-up studies* seemed the most pertinent.

The final choice of search words for the Medline database in the order intended to be tried were *breast neoplasm; mastectomy, segmental; follow-up studies.*

Set	Search	Results
1	explode *breast neoplasm/*	16 631
2	*mastectomy, segmental/*	478
3	1 or 2	16 649
4	*follow-up studies*	42 140
5	3 and 4	872
6	limit 5 to English language	783
7	*family practice/*	5543
8	explode *primary healthcare/*	4878
9	7 or 8	9864
10	6 and 9	4

Once the three chosen search terms had been keyed in and the 872 references resulting restricted to those in English language in set 6, the search was focused on the secondary care setting in line with the original question. However, keying in *secondary care* gave a selection of branch terms in the MeSH headings of which *family practice* and then *health services research* were the most popular options. The option *family practice* was selected as being the real setting of interest despite the original wording of the question, and the term *primary healthcare* was included too to reduce the chances of missing relevant papers. This identified four references in set 10. Browsing through the abstracts found one reference of particular interest:

▶ Grunfeld E, Gray A, Mant D, Yudkin P, Adewuyi-Dalton R, Coyle D, Cole D, Stewart J, Fitzpatrick R, Vessey M (1999) Follow-up of breast cancer in primary care vs specialist care: results of an economic evaluation. *British Journal of Cancer.* **79**(7–8): 1227–33.

Another way of tracking references and trying to make sure you are not missing any relevant ones, or opening a new avenue if you are stuck in your search down a blind alley, is to look down the list of references given in a relevant published paper to give you new ideas about which other MeSH headings you might explore.

In this case the searcher was aware of a paper published by Grunfeld *et al.* in 1996 and so changed databases to search Medline 1993–1996. However, repeating the search strategy outlined above failed to identify this paper. The reason for the omission turned out to be that the term was written as *follow up* without a hyphen in the title of the 1996 paper (Grunfeld E, Mant D, Yudkin P, *et al.* (1996) Routine follow up of breast cancer in primary care: randomised trial. *BMJ.* **313**: 665–9) whereas the term *follow-up* in the MeSH heading had a hyphen. Searching on *follow up* without a hyphen identified the reference; the two Grunfeld *et al.* papers of 1995 and 1996 were indexed differently.

Searching by yourself

Now you do it – work through an example by yourself.

1 Take any one (or all) of the four problems which interests you most – whether health education on smoking is worth doing, the problem of the mother wanting to know if the likely improvement to her child's eczema warrants the efforts involved in minimising house dust at home, whether it is

cost-effective to screen all diabetics for microalbuminuria, or if patients who have had a lumpectomy for breast cancer are best followed up in secondary care. Adapt the problem(s) to your own circumstances. The idea of this exercise is that you will run a search on a similar question (or questions) to the ones already described so that you can follow the procedures laid out in this book for guidance, but adapted to your own situation so that it is more relevant to you. Conducting your own version of the search will give you more confidence that you can do a literature search yourself. Write in your own words what your perspective of the problem is:

2 Frame the words of your question to address that problem – the words you use in the question should vary from any presented in this book as the angle of the problem and the focus of the question should relate to your own circumstances. Write in your own words what the question is:

3 Choose up to five key words and put them in order of priority:

4 Undertake a search for the evidence to answer that problem. If possible go to your medical library and book time with a medical librarian and the computerised search facilities there. If the library has Cochrane and Medline searching facilities, use the Cochrane database first and then Medline.

Photocopy pages 58–60 if you undertake this exercise for more than one example question.

Cochrane search

▶ Write down how you will use your key words to search the Cochrane database. Which one, two or three words will you key in first? Then, which words will you add, and in what order, to narrow the focus of your search?

▶ How did the search go? How many 'hits' did you obtain from the Cochrane database?
  – systematic reviews on the Cochrane Database of Systematic Reviews (CDSR):
    (i) number of reviews =
    (ii) number of protocols =
  – controlled trials on the Cochrane Controlled Trials Register (CCTR) =
  – abstracts on the Database of Abstracts of Reviews of Effectiveness (DARE) =

▶ Write down up to five sets of details of articles that seem relevant to your question, giving article titles, authors' names, year of publication, volume of journal/source and page details so that you can obtain the original papers if you should wish to. Print off the abstracts if you have the facilities to do so.

Medline search

▶ Write down how you will use your key words to search the Medline database. Which one, two or three words will you key in first? Then, which words will you add, and in what order, to narrow the focus of your search?

▶ Begin your search and key the words in, exploding, combining and modifying the search according to the order of key words you have just specified and the numbers of papers you obtain at each stage. Go back to the instructions about using Medline and work through the examples and helpful suggestions if you have difficulties doing your own search.

▶ How did the search go? Print off the results of the search in the same way as the tables given as examples earlier listed the stages of the search, the modifications and the numbers of papers identified from the key words. If you cannot print the results off the screen, copy them down over the page under the sub-headings 'Set', 'Search' and 'Results' as in the example tables.

Set	Search	Results
1		

▶ When you get down to less than 20 or so articles, scroll through the abstracts on the screen and print off the details of the ones that seem most relevant. Write down up to five sets of details of articles that seem relevant, giving article titles, authors' names, year of publication, volume of journal/source and page details.

▶ If you have still not obtained any relevant evidence you have a choice of trying other databases, or following up references given in papers with content nearest to your field of enquiry, or contacting experts named as authors or investigators to find out if there is work in press or other publications you have missed, or any other pertinent information.

You should not expect to find exactly the same details as in the examples given earlier as not only will you have modified the problem, the linked question and the search strategy to fit your own circumstances, but the details of publications held on the Cochrane and Medline databases will have changed over time.

▼

Choose a question that is important to you and your colleagues at work and where
changes in practice will be possible.

► STAGE 3

Frame your own question and search for the evidence

Now that you have learnt the theory behind doing a search and have seen how other health professionals like you have framed their questions and searched for the evidence, you should be ready to shape your own question and find the best available evidence that exists.

1 Think about a problem at work which you consider would be an appropriate topic for this exercise. Consult others at work, do they think it is a problem too? Is it an important issue for them and do they think you would be spending your time wisely searching for evidence about best practice? Is there likely to be a change that you could make which would bring benefits to you, colleagues or patients, or result in a saving of resources? As this book is considering how to improve clinical effectiveness you should choose a clinical topic in this instance, but another time you might choose to search for evidence on a management issue. What is the problem you have chosen to investigate? Write it down here:

Who else did you consult before deciding on this problem?

What sort of changes at work do you have in mind that might be possible to put into action, depending on what evidence you find?

2 Frame the words of your question which address that problem. Build up the question as described previously, being as specific as possible, but not so specific that you narrow your field of enquiry and eliminate possible options that might be appropriate, such as novel types of interventions. Include the purpose of the question, what it is about, the setting, the population and the outcome(s). Write in your own words what the question is:

Are there any subsidiary questions?

Have you discussed the question with anyone else? If so, with whom?

3 Choose up to five key words and put them in order of priority:

Are you satisfied that these key words reflect all the essential ingredients of your original problem and capture the essence of the question?

4 Undertake a search for the evidence to answer the question. If possible go to your medical library and book time with a medical librarian and the computerised search facilities there. If the library has Cochrane and Medline searching facilities, try the Cochrane database first and then Medline.

Cochrane search

▶ Write down how you will use your key words to search the Cochrane database. Which one, two or three words will you key in first? Then, which words will you add, and in what order, to narrow the focus of your search?

▶ How did the search go? How many 'hits' did you obtain from the Cochrane database?
  – systematic reviews on the Cochrane Database of Systematic Reviews (CDSR):
    (i) number of reviews =
    (ii) number of protocols =
  – controlled trials on the Cochrane Controlled Trials Register (CCTR) =
  – abstracts on the Database of Abstracts of Reviews of Effectiveness (DARE) =

▶ Write down up to five sets of details of articles that seem relevant to your question, giving article titles, authors' names, year of publication, volume of journal/source and page details. Print off the abstracts of these articles if you are able to do so. Obtain copies of the original papers.

Medline search

▶ Write down how you will use your key words to search the Medline database. Which one, two or three words will you key in first? Then, which words will you add, and in what order, to narrow the focus of your search?

▶ Begin your search and key the words in, exploding, combining and modifying the search according to the order of key words you have just specified and the numbers of papers you obtain at each stage.

▶ How did the search go? Print off the results of the search in the same way as the tables given as examples earlier listed the stages of the search, the modifications and the numbers of papers identified from the key words. If you cannot print the results off the screen, copy them down here under the sub-headings 'Set', 'Search' and 'Results' as in the example tables.

Set	Search	Results
1		

▶ When you get down to less than 20 or so articles, scroll through the abstracts on the screen and print off the details of the ones that seem most relevant. Write down up to five sets of details of articles that seem relevant, giving article titles, authors' names, year of publication, volume of journal/source and page details.

► If you have still not obtained any relevant evidence you have a choice of trying other databases, or following up references given in papers with content nearest to your field of enquiry, or contacting experts named as authors or investigators to find out if there is work in press or other publications you have missed, or any other pertinent information.

Save your search on a floppy disc before logging off so that you can come back to where you were if you want to continue to modify the search upon later reflection.

Appraise the evidence

Now that you have extracted the publications that seem most relevant to your own question from your search, the next steps are to decide how much reliance you can put on their contents and how far you can extrapolate from those papers to your own circumstances. This will involve deciding whether the studies described in the papers were well conducted or flawed, whether the population and setting studied were similar enough to your own circumstances for the results to be generalisable to your population or setting, whether sufficient people or things were studied for the results to be representative of larger numbers, and how you will weigh one paper against another if they report conflicting results or conclusions.

Critical appraisal is the assessment of evidence by systematically reviewing its relevance, validity and results to specific situations.

Critical appraisal:

► identifies the strengths and weaknesses of a research paper
► develops a better understanding of scientific principles and research methodology
► increases capability to understand to what extent published literature is applicable to other circumstances.

The meaning of different research methods and terms

Bias

Systematic deviation of the results from the true results due to the way(s) in which the study was carried out.

Confidence intervals

This describes the degree of confidence that can be placed on any statistical result. It describes the range of results from the subjects or things studied within which the investigator is 95% certain that the true population mean lies (the usual level of confidence chosen).

Confounder

A factor, other than the variables under study, which is not controlled for and which distorts the results causing a spurious association.

Controlled trial

As for a randomised controlled trial (see relevant entry) without the randomisation element.

A controlled trial detects associations between an intervention and an outcome but does not rule out the possibility that the association was caused by an unrecognised third factor linking both the intervention and the outcome.

Controls

The subjects in a (randomised) controlled trial who are (randomly) allocated to receive either placebo, no treatment or the standard treatment.

Cost-effectiveness analysis (CEA)

Compares the effectiveness of two interventions with the same treatment objectives. Competing interventions are compared in terms of costs per unit of consequence. Consequences may vary but are measured in monetary terms.

Cost-benefit analysis (CBA)

Compares the incremental costs and benefits of a programme. Measures both costs and benefits in monetary values and calculates net monetary gains or losses (presented as a cost-benefit ratio).

Cost-minimisation analysis (CMA)

Compares the costs of alternative treatments that have identical outcomes.

Cost-utility analysis (CUA)

Measures the effects of alternative interventions in terms of a combination of life expectancy and quality of life, using utility measures such as quality-adjusted life years (QALYs) and may present relative costs per QALY.

Efficacy

The extent to which an intervention produces a beneficial result under ideal conditions. Preferably based on an RCT.

Effectiveness

The extent to which an intervention does what it is intended to do for a defined population.

Hawthorne effect

The influence of knowledge of the study on behaviour. The effect of being in a study on the persons being studied.

Incidence

The numbers or proportion of new cases of a disease or condition occurring within a population over a given period of time.

Intention to treat analysis

This is a quantitative estimate of the benefit of a therapy in the population being studied derived from comparing control and treatment groups.

Numbers needed to treat (NNT) are being cited in published papers increasingly commonly. You need to know the characteristics of the population being studied, the disease and its severity, the treatment and its duration, the comparator and the outcomes.

Meta-analysis

This is a method of combining two or more studies to obtain information about larger numbers of subjects. Inclusion criteria should be clearly stated in the method to enable different studies to be considered together. It should appear reasonable to treat the sum of the different studies as one whole and that like is being combined with like.

Observational study

There are several types of study where the subjects are observed over time and the experiences are recorded or reported.

A cohort study is one where two similar groups of people who do not have the disease or condition under study are observed prospectively over a predetermined period to see the effects of one group being exposed to an already established suspected risk factor (such as cigarette smoking) and the other group not being so exposed.

A cross-sectional survey gathers information about subjects or things in a study population at one point in time or over a relatively short period.

Odds Ratio (OR)

A measure of treatment effectiveness. The probability of an event happening as opposed to it not happening. An OR of 1 means that the effects of treatment are no different from no treatment. If the OR is greater than (or less than) 1, it means that the effects of treatment are more (or less) than those of the control group.

Placebo

An inert substance that is given to control subjects in trials.

Power

Sample sizes should be calculated before the study design is finalised to determine the numbers needed to be likely to detect a sufficient effect from the study intervention, so as to be sure that the effect did not occur by chance alone. The power calculation predicts the number needing to be studied to detect an effect at least at the level of 95% significance. This is the level of certainty that is equal to or less than a one in 20 risk that the effect occurred by chance and was not due to an intervention or event being studied.

Prevalence

The proportion of 'cases' within a specified population at a given time.

Probability

Probabilities are often written as p values in published reports where p stands for probability. It is a measure of how likely an outcome is. This lies between 0 (where an event will never happen) and 1.0 (where it will definitely occur).

The p value is a guide to the likelihood that the outcome measured occurred by chance or was due to the intervention or event that the study was designed to measure.

A significant p value is one where the likelihood is that the effect or outcome occurred as a result of the intervention or event being studied, and did not occur by chance. The most common convention is to decide arbitrarily on a one in 20 risk of being wrong about the direct causal relationship between the intervention or event and the outcome; that is, the risk that the outcome occurred by chance. This can be described as '$p = 0.05$', 'at the 5% significance level' or as a '5 in 100 probability' that the outcome occurred by chance. If written as '$p < 0.05$' there is less than 5 in 100 risk of the outcome having happened by chance. Smaller p values give increased confidence in the test results; for example $p < 0.001$ indicates that the probability that the outcome occurred by chance is less than one in a thousand. The level of significance the investigators choose should depend on the importance of being right about the intervention/outcome relationship, and the numbers in the populations being studied.

Sometimes investigators get carried away, testing every bit of data in their study to see if they can dredge up some significant results. This is very bad practice because even a short questionnaire can yield hundreds of combinations of possibilities if each question has several alternative categories of answers, for example age might be subdivided into nine decades. If a significance test was applied to all the possible combinations of answers looking for potential links and 200 tests of significance were tried, for example, you would expect ten tests erroneously to indicate statistical significance where the outcome(s) had occurred by chance (that is, 5 in 100 risk $\times 2 = 10$). So the arbitrary $p < 0.05$ test of assumed significance is not cut-and-dried proof that an outcome is directly attributable to an intervention – it is just a good indicator of significance.

Publication bias

Results are more likely to be published if the results are positive rather than negative. Thus, it may appear that treatments have more positive results than is actually the case.

Randomised controlled trial (RCT)

Randomisation is necessary to minimise and, hopefully, eliminate selection bias. This is the type of study design which is most likely to give you a true result because only one section of the subjects or things in the trial are exposed to the intervention or factor being studied. The subjects or things are randomly allocated either to the group exposed to the intervention or to the control group who are not intentionally exposed to that intervention. The experiences and outcomes of both groups are compared to see if they are significantly different according to statistical tests. Sometimes the design includes more than two comparative groups.

Using the randomised controlled trial method distributes unsuspected biological variables equally between the two groups, as well as any other external factors of which you are unaware. Both the subject and control groups will be exposed to these unrecognised external influences (called confounding factors) and any differences in outcomes between the two groups should be attributable to the intervention being studied.

When the term 'randomised' is stated there should be some information in the method as to how this randomisation process was carried out to minimise any external influences from interfering with the random allocation of subjects or things to different arms of the study.

If a trial is 'double blind', neither the clinician/investigator giving the treatment or analysing the results, nor the person receiving it, should know whether they are in the treatment or the control group. In a 'single' blind study, either the clinician or the subject knows what treatment the subject is receiving.

Relative risk

Relative risk is calculated by taking the ratio between two measures of risk. If there is no difference between two groups the risk ratio is '1' as the risks in each group are the same. A risk ratio greater than '1' shows the outcome in the study group to be better than that for controls.

The risk ratio is the proportion of the group at risk in one group divided by the proportion at risk in a second group. The risk ratio is a measure of relative risk.

Reliability

A reliable method is one which produces repeatable results.

Sensitivity of test

The true positive rate of a diagnostic test, that is, how often the test misses people with the disease.

Sensitivity analysis

Tests the robustness of the results of an economic analysis by varying the underlying assumptions around which there is uncertainty.

Specificity of test

The true negative rate of a diagnostic test, that is, how often the test indicates people as having the disease when they do not.

Statistically significant

By convention taken to be at the 5% level (p<0.05). This means that the observed result would occur by chance in only one in 20 cases (*see* Probability).

Systematic review

Systematic reviews of randomised controlled trials provide the highest level of evidence of the effectiveness of treatments – preventative, therapeutic and rehabilitatory treatments (as described in the section on hierarchy of evidence, pp 43–4).

Validity

A valid method is one which measures what it sets out to measure.

Reading a paper

Reading and evaluating a paper is mainly about applying common sense. Traditionally, critical appraisal of the literature has been made to seem like a difficult science for the elite, rather than a basic skill that any health professional can readily learn and apply to their own situation.

If you read the summary of a research study overleaf and answer the questions you will soon discover for yourself some of the common flaws in published studies, sometimes even those in respected peer-reviewed journals where the mistakes were not noted by the researchers or publication team.

In general you should consider whether:

► the paper is relevant to your own practice
► the research question is well defined
► any definitions are unambiguous
► the aim(s) and/or objective(s) of the study are clearly stated
► the design and methodology are appropriate for the aim(s) of the study
► the measuring instruments seem to be reliable; that is, different observers at different points in time would arrive at the same outcome
► the measuring instruments seem to be valid; that is, the investigator is actually measuring that which she/he intends to measure

- the sampling method is clear
- the results relate to the aim(s) and objective(s) of the study
- the results seem to be robust and justifiable
- the results can be generalised to your own circumstances
- there are any biases in the method of the study
- there are biases in the results, such as non-reporting of drop-outs from the study
- the conclusion is valid
- you have any other concerns about the study.

Specifically you should look at:

- where the study was done and who are the authors
- the study design: how were the subjects and controls selected, were they randomised and if so how, what were the outcome measures, were the outcome measures clinically relevant, are the sample numbers appropriate?
- the results: are the numbers of drop-outs and non-respondents reported, are all subjects accounted for, is the statistical analysis explained, are the results clearly presented?
- the discussion and conclusions: does the report describe the study's limitations, are the conclusions supported by the results?

Critical appraisal of a published paper or report of a study

1 The aim(s) and /or objective(s) of the study should be stated clearly.

  - The aim should state the purpose of the study succinctly and specifically. It should be set in the context of information that is already known from previously published literature.

  - The reasons for, and need to carry out, the study should be justified in the introduction of the paper.

> ► There should be a clear route built up from the aim to the conclusion flowing from the explanation of why a particular study design, population and setting were selected, to the results reported, the discussion and interpretation and final conclusion(s).

2 The methodology should be appropriate for the aim of the study.

> ► Quantitative and qualitative design techniques are complementary. A good quantitative survey will be based on prior qualitative work to determine what are appropriate questions to ask in the questionnaire or interview schedule. A randomised controlled trial may be a gold standard quantitative study design, but a qualitative method will most probably be needed to report people's observations, reflections and judgements.
> ► As a generalisation, prospective recording is more likely to be accurate than retrospective recall.
> ► A sample of a population should be selected for study which is as representative as possible of the whole population.
> ► A setting should be chosen for a study which is as representative as possible of the setting of the total population to which the results of the study will be extrapolated.
> ► The sample size should be justified by a *power calculation* determined prior to starting the study based on the expected findings.
> ► There should be a method for increasing the response rate to as near as possible an ideal of 100% of the subjects included in the study.
> ► Details of any measurement or intervention should be as specific as possible, and transparently valid and reliable.
> ► A good study design will include a method to validate the questionnaire, rating scale or results obtained.
> ► It is always a bonus to see an original questionnaire even if only in an abbreviated form, to be able to judge

for yourself the validity of the questions used in the study.

▶ The statistical methods should be described so that when the results are reported readers can check the statistical calculations and understand how the results were derived from the original data, if they wish.

3 The results should be robust, justified and related to the objectives of the study.

▶ The results should be simple to understand. It should be obvious where the results have come from and they should not seem to have been plucked out of thin air. Graphs and tables help to avoid strings of numbers and percentages.

▶ Statistically significant results should be presented in a conventional way or explained with full references if less well known statistical tests are used.

▶ Percentages should add up to 100% and if they do not there should be some explanation to account for the missing numbers. It should be clear where and whether subjects have not sent back the questionnaire, have left a particular question blank or given a 'don't know' response.

▶ If the results obtained from the subjects are fairly crude, such as when people are asked to estimate their answers or recall happenings in the distant past, the result should be given as whole numbers or to one decimal place, rather than given as several decimal places which might look more scientific to the casual reader.

▶ The written contents of a research paper should be in their correct places. Bits of method should not crop up afresh in the results, nor should discussion be interspersed in the results. The flow of the paper should be logical and build up to a justifiable conclusion. Anything otherwise is confusion and muddle.

▶ A low response rate may mean that the results from the sample of the population studied are not likely to be representative of the whole population. The further you regress from a 100% response rate the more likely it is that you have missed people or things that would give your results a different slant. As a very rough guide, a response rate of 70% seems generally to be regarded as reasonable for a topic where the results are not going to have dire consequences if they are wrong. But if the study was a trial of drug therapy where people's lives might be at stake if the research results and conclusions were wrong, anything less than a 100% response rate might be unacceptable.

4 Any biases in the design and execution of the study should be minimised and their likely influences acknowledged and explained.

  ▸ Good response rates are important because responders may have different characteristics from those of non-responders.
  ▸ There may be confounding factors present. These are so-far undetected influences that were not measured or recorded in the course of the study, that were actually wholly or partly responsible for causing the changes or results reported. There are often cultural changes with time outside the study and beyond the control of those undertaking the investigation. For instance, if a famous celebrity claimed benefits for a new treatment that was being studied, many more people would suddenly believe they had received the same benefits and the outcomes being studied at that time would be distorted. Opting for *randomised controlled trials* avoids the influence of confounding factors.
  ▸ The potential and actual biases of the study should be openly described and their likely effects discussed in the Discussion section of the paper. Readers should then be able to make up their own minds about the relative importance of each bias on the results and how much the biases prejudice the extrapolation of the results to the readers' own situations.

5 Is the conclusion valid?

   ▶ The conclusion is often found in the Discussion section of a paper when there is no separate Conclusion section.
   ▶ The conclusions of the results should not hinge on probability test results. The significance of the results claimed should make sense from clinical and common sense perspectives too. For example, an intervention might claim that it is significantly better than another at increasing small children's height by 0.1 inches. But if, clinically, this difference is inconsequential, then the benefits of the treatment claiming to be superior are not proven by the positive significant result.
   ▶ The conclusion(s) should not make any claims that have not been justified previously in the report of the study.
   ▶ No new information should suddenly crop up in the conclusions that was not previously cited in the method, results or other section.
   ▶ It should be clear what the main findings mean and the implications for current practice or future developments.
   ▶ The results of the current study should be compared and contrasted with others reported elsewhere and any discrepancies interpreted and discussed.

6 Any other concerns about the study.

   ▶ Conflicts of interest should be stated, such as the sponsorship of the study by a manufacturer of the medication tested in the study.
   ▶ Look for any omissions in any section of the report. Think whether the implications from any contrary results seem to have been considered in full or glossed over.

Examples

Critically appraise this example – a summary report of a research study.

1 An investigation of the use of sunscreens in the United Kingdom

Summary

Aim: To investigate the use of sunscreens in children.

Method: A postal questionnaire was sent out to all 942 members of Women's Institutes throughout the Scottish Isles, asking them about the frequency of the use of high-factor sunscreens applied to their children (please contact the author for a copy of the questionnaire). Questionnaires were anonymous to ensure confidentiality. An article was placed in the Women's Institute newsletter to prompt non-responders.

Results: 356 women replied (85% response rate; average age 56 + SD 16.4298 years). 290 stated that they bought factor 10 or higher sunscreen. 89 preferred the scent-free version ($p < 0.1$). 350 women thought that the government should subsidise the cost of sunscreens as they were too expensive ($p < 0.0001$). The presence of a melanoma should be treated as a criminal offence and the sufferer fined for not having used sufficient sunscreen, as a contribution to the costs of the ensuing NHS treatment.

Conclusion: If the government were to subsidise the cost of buying high-factor sunscreens, uptake would be increased and the frequency of melanomas or other skin cancers would fall.

Source of funding: Nibblea Suncreams.

Conflict of interest: None.

Chambers R (1998) *J Evidence-Based Spoof.* **3:** 12.

Consider the following challenges

Write down your answers then read the author's opinion below:

1 Are the aim(s) and/or objective(s) of the study clearly stated?

2 Is the methodology appropriate for the aim(s) of the study?

3 Do the results relate to the aims(s) and/or objective(s) of the study? Are the results robust and justified?

4 Are there any biases in the design and execution of the study?

5 Is the conclusion valid?

6 Are there any other concerns about the study?

Critique of the summary report: use of sunscreens in the United Kingdom

1 Are the aim(s) and/or objective(s) of the study clearly stated?

The aim is not very specific. If the focus of the conclusion on cost of sunscreens and the impact of sunscreens on the frequency of cancers were intended as the purpose of the study then the aim has been expressed incorrectly.

2 Is the methodology appropriate for the aim(s) of the study?

No, no, no! There is already confusion as the aim and conclusions are so far apart, but working on the premise of the aim stated in the summary of the study given:

▸ the population chosen for study is inappropriate as children of Women's Institute members probably range in age from 1 to 60 years old; this can be deduced from the subject's average age being 56 years and the standard deviation (SD) of 16.4 years indicating that about two-thirds of the population studied are between 40 and 70 years (that is, $56 - 16.4$ years = 40 years to $56 + 16.4$ years = 70 years)

- ▶ the Scottish Isles setting is in a part of the United Kingdom that would be expected to have relatively low amounts and strength of ultraviolet rays, and results from this setting cannot necessarily be generalised elsewhere
- ▶ members of Women's Institutes living in the Scottish Isles whilst the study was in progress had not necessarily lived there all their lives; so if the geographical area was important the mothers do not have uniform histories of where they lived when younger, and their children may have lived apart from their mothers at any time previously
- ▶ the differing age range of the children means that some mothers' reports will relate to children under the age of 18 years currently receiving modern types of high-factor sunscreens, and others will relate to middle-aged children who may or may not have had old-fashioned creams applied a varying number of years previously; high-factor sunscreens did not exist at the time the study began
- ▶ there is no logic in choosing Women's Institute members as the population group to be studied – it may introduce a further bias if it were shown that members were more likely to be part of a more affluent section of society than the general population as a whole and therefore more likely to take holidays abroad where the sunshine was more powerful and potentially damaging
- ▶ mothers' recall of the frequency of use of suncreams applied to children up to 50 years before is unlikely to be accurate
- ▶ anonymous questionnaires that do not bear a code number make chasing up of individual non-respondents impossible – an article placed in a newsletter is unlikely to be an effective method of encouraging non-responders to reply.

3 Do the results relate to the aim(s) and/or objective(s) of the study? Are the results robust and justified?

It is obvious that the results are inaccurate and meaningless. Also:

- ▸ the response rate was very low at 38% (356/942), not 85% as stated
- ▸ the results, such as the information about costs of sunscreens, are not related to the data that would have arisen from the study method described
- ▸ it is ridiculous to give the standard deviation (SD) to four decimal places when the average age is given as a whole number
- ▸ a probability of < 0.1 is not significant and no such conclusions can be drawn about a proportion of the population studied preferring the scent-free version
- ▸ results should be factual and not offer interpretations, as here where the government is encouraged to treat the presence of melanomas as a criminal offence
- ▸ the results cannot be generalised.

4 Are there any biases in the design and execution of the study?

The study is riddled with biases from start to finish. Many have been described already, such as:

- ▸ the nature of the population
- ▸ that retrospective recall of information is likely to be poor
- ▸ the poor response rate
- ▸ the changing nature of commercially available sunscreens over time throughout the study
- ▸ the fact that the conclusion does not relate to the rest of the study, which implies that the whole purpose of the study may have been to prove that sunscreens should be subsidised and that the design and reporting of the study might be biased to that end.

5 Is the conclusion valid?

No it is not. It does not follow from the rest of the report and is not related to the original aim.

6 Are there are any other concerns about the study?

Although the author of this report states that there was no conflict of interest, the sponsorship of the study by a manufacturer of suncreams should alert readers to scrutinise the report even more carefully than usual for possible biases.

▼

Remember that sometimes the evidence can be misleading.

2 An investigation of prisoners' health compared with that of the general population

Critically appraise this second example – an unpublished report of a research study. Answer the following challenges, as before – write down your answers then read the author's opinion:

1 Are the aim(s) and/or objective(s) of the study clearly stated?

2 Is the methodology appropriate for the aim(s) of the study?

3 Do the results relate to the aims(s) and/or objective(s) of the study? Are the results robust and justified?

4 Are there any biases in the design and execution of the study?

5 Is the conclusion valid?

6 Are there any other concerns about the study?

Introduction: Recent work has shown that prisoners are disadvantaged in terms of their social background, their health status and the quality of healthcare they receive (Smith 1984; Walmsley *et al.* 1992). Research carried out in Bedford prison (Martin *et al.* 1984) found that prisoners had tended to neglect their health before reception into prison and 46% had active medical problems at admission.

Many of the people sent to prison have mental health problems. Gunn and others (1991) found that 37% of sentenced prisoners sampled from prisons in England and Wales had a psychiatric disorder, 2% of whom were suffering from a psychosis that was being inadequately treated and required transfer to hospital. A further 15% were thought to require additional treatment at the prison for their psychiatric problems.

The suicide rate amongst prisoners is several times that of their peers in the community and is rising disproportionately to the increase in the prison population (Dooley 1990). In 1992–93 (Wool 1994), 27 male prisoners committed suicide and in addition there were open verdicts on ten other males who died. The number of recorded incidents of self-injury is also rising steadily – 2612 prisoners were reported to have injured themselves on 3281 occasions in 1992–93 (Wool 1994).

A recent review of prisoners' physical health (Adam 1994) reported an increased incidence of alcohol problems, epilepsy, peptic ulceration, hypertension, hepatitis B infection, tuberculosis and self-neglect (skin infections, caries). Alcoholism is ten times more common amongst new prisoners than in the general community and 86% of new prisoners smoke (Martin *et al.* 1984).

This study set out to compare lifestyle habits of inmates in six prisons in the West Midlands with general population norms and measured prisoners' general health using the SF36 health measure (Jenkinson *et al.* 1993).

Method: Between 50 and 61 prisoners in each of the six prisons were surveyed between March and August 1994. Prisoners were interviewed in private rooms by the research associate. All prisoners thought to offer a potential security risk and those residing in punishment blocks were excluded from the study. Fifty prisoners were recruited in all establishments except one prison where 61 prisoners were chosen to allow sufficient sampling of the remand as well as the convicted men, and a second prison where 60 men were selected when two blocks of prisoners were demarcated for the study.

The method of selection varied according to individual prison procedures. In three prisons, clerical staff did not allow access to lists of prisoners' names and prisoners were recruited by a volunteer system. In the fourth prison all 60 inmates on education and physical education courses were interviewed. In the fifth and sixth prisons, every tenth inmate was selected from the list of inmates. Prisoners who refused or could not be interviewed were replaced by volunteers.

The interviews were conducted in a private room in which only the researcher and inmate were present, or a quiet corner of a large room. The inmate was assured that any information given was confidential to the research team and that a report would not identify any individual prisoners. All questions were asked by the interviewer so that literacy was not required.

The interviewer asked questions about lifestyle, and administered the SF36 survey form (Saudi Arabian version) (Ware and Sherbourne 1992).

The question schedule was piloted on ten prisoners before the main study began. Questions were amended accordingly. The prisoners participating in the pilot survey were excluded from the prison population selected for the survey.

A Minitab statistical package was used for processing the data and analysing the results.

Results: Thirty-six of the total 381 prisoners invited to be interviewed did not attend because they were unwilling, had appointments elsewhere, were thought by prison staff to be unsuitable for interview for security reasons, were confined to the punishment blocks or refused to be studied.

The mean ages of prisoners interviewed are shown in Table 1. All were convicted prisoners except 24 of the 61 surveyed in one prison, who were on remand.

Table 1: Age of prisoners interviewed in the six prisons studied

Prison code number	Mean age of subjects (standard deviation)*
P1 (n = 61)	18.2 (1.5)
P2 (n = 60)	16.1 (0.9)
P3 (n = 50)	32.4 (11.1)
P4 (n = 50)	27.4 (6.5)
P5 (n = 50)	32.1 (9.9)
P6 (n = 50)	19.7 (0.9)

*Age ranges have not been given so as to preserve prison anonymity.

Table 2: Current smoking habits of inmates in the six prisons

Prison code number	Percentage of prisoners who were current smokers
P1 ($n = 61$)	90
P2 ($n = 60$)	82
P3 ($n = 50$)	82
P4 ($n = 50$)	88
P5 ($n = 50$)	60
P6 ($n = 50$)	90

Table 2 describes prisoners' smoking habits in gaol. Smoking was as common amongst young offenders as older adults. Less than five per cent of prisoners who had previously not been smoking had started smoking during their time in prison. There was a slight tendency for smokers to report that they smoked more heavily since coming to prison.

The majority of inmates (91%) in all six prisons exercised on three days per week or more. Six per cent of prisoners never exercised in five of the six prisons. Forty-six per cent of prisoners interviewed reported that they exercised more during their time in prison compared to when they were 'outside', 15% thought the frequency was about the same, and 38% thought they exercised less in prison.

All 321 prisoners who completed the questionnaire about lifestyle also answered the SF36 health survey. Table 3 gives the mean score for the eight variables of the SF36 and norms for a comparable group from the general population matched for age and sex, taken from Jenkinson *et al.* (1993). Prisoner means that were statistically different from general population norms are indicated in Table 3.

Mean SF36 scores for prisoners of all six prisons were significantly worse than general population norms for social functioning ($p < 0.001$ in all cases), mental health ($p < 0.001$ in five out of six prisons, and $p < 0.05$ in P4) and pain dimensions; in five out of six prisons, inmates had mean SF36

Table 3: Mean scores for eight variables of SF36 for prisoners from the six prisons and norms for a comparable group matched for age and sex, taken from Jenkinson *et al.* (1993)

Prison code number	Physical function	Social function	Physical limits	Emotional limits	Mental health	Energy/ vitality	Pain	General health
P1								
Age/sex match	92.8	90.2	91.8	82.9	74.8	66.4	86.6	72.0
Prisoners	97.5*	78.9**	80.0**	77.0	65.3*	57.3**	75.4**	67.3
P2								
Age/sex match	92.8	90.2	91.8	82.9	74.8	66.4	86.6	72.0
Prisoners	97.1	81.6**	73.8**	81.7	63.5**	49.3**	75.3**	68.4
P3								
Age/sex match	91.9	90.4	90.4	85.4	75.5	64.7	85.9	73.9
Prisoners	91.8	70.7**	78.5**	66.6**	65.2**	54.7**	67.7**	68.5
P4								
Age/sex match	93.1	90.7	91.6	85.1	75.3	65.2	86.8	74.3
Prisoners	93.7	72.9**	85.5	74.6*	69.4*	60.5	72.2**	66.1*
P5								
Age/sex match	90.2	86.6	86.0	80.2	71.5	58.8	80.8	74.7
Prisoners	81.2**	64.9**	76.0*	58.5**	53.5**	42.3**	54.5**	63.6**
P6								
Age/sex match	92.8	90.2	91.8	82.9	74.8	66.4	86.6	72.0
Prisoners	96.3	76.7**	84.0*	86.0	66.6**	59.4*	77.9*	66.9

Prisoner means that are statistically significant in comparison with the group matched for age and sex are shown by *($p < 0.05$) or **($p < 0.001$).

scores that were significantly worse than age and sex matched norms for physical limitations and vitality.

Discussion: This survey proves that prisoners have worse health and well-being according to a comparison with the general public using the SF36 scale.

The volunteers used in place of those prisoners who refused or were not allowed to participate in the study were suitable replacements as the interviewer picked subjects who worked in the same workplace or lived in the same prison wings instead. The chocolate gratuity received by prisoners who had satisfied the interviewer's questions was not considered to have biased the results.

Prisoners' exercise habits compared favourably with those of doctors, where 22% have been found never to exercise and only 16% to exercise at least twice per week (Chambers 1992). Far more of the prisoner subjects smoked compared to a third of adults in the general population (Health Education Authority 1989).

The SF36 scale is reliable, valid and acceptable. The numbers of statistically significant differences were startling compared to the general public's norms.

Conclusions: The general public is healthier than prisoners in the United Kingdom.

References for the paper:

Adam S (1994) *Learning Across the Walls: the prison service and the NHS.* King's Fund Centre, London.

Chambers R (1992) Health and lifestyle of general practitioners and teachers. *Occup Med.* **42**: 69–78.

Dooley E (1990) Prison suicide in England and Wales, 1972–87. *Br J Psych.* **156**: 40–5.

Gunn J, Maden A and Swinton M (1991) Treatment needs of prisoners with psychiatric disorders. *BMJ.* **303**: 338–41.

Health Education Authority (1989) *Strategic Plan 1990–95*. Health Education Authority, London.

Jenkinson C, Coulter A and Wright L (1993) Short form 36 (SF36) health survey questionnaire: normative data for adults of working age. *BMJ*. **306**: 1437–40.

Martin E, Colebrook M and Gray A (1984) Health of prisoners admitted to and discharged from Bedford prison. *BMJ*. **289**: 965–7.

Smith R (1984) *Prison Health Care*. British Medical Association, London.

Walmsley R, Howard L and White S (1992) *National Prison Survey 1991*. HMSO, London.

Ware JE and Sherbourne CD (1992) The MOS 36-item short-form health survey (SF36) 1: conceptual framework and item selection. *Med Care*. **30**: 473–83.

Wool R (1994) *Report of the Director of Health Care for Prisoners. April 1992–March 1993*. HM Prison Service.

Critique of the report: an investigation of how healthy prisoners are compared with the general population

This critique picks out main points and is not intended to be comprehensive. The report concerns a real study that was carried out by the author but has been adulterated to illustrate learning points.

1 Are the aim(s) and/or objective(s) of the study clearly stated?

Yes, they are stated at the end of the introduction. But the bulk of the material set out in the introduction refers to the mental health of prisoners, whereas the aims imply that the study is mainly concerned with prisoners' physical health.

2 Is the methodology appropriate for the aim(s) of the study?

- ▸ The use of an interviewer for questioning prisoners seems appropriate as a considerable number of prisoners might be expected to be illiterate.
- ▸ There is no power calculation or indication of whether 50 to 61 inmates from each prison were valid sample sizes.
- ▸ The Saudi Arabian version of the SF36 might be inappropriate for measuring the health of a British population.
- ▸ It was good that a pilot study was undertaken to test the questionnaire and that those subjects were excluded from the main study.
- ▸ There is insufficient detail about recruitment and selection of prisons and subjects, administration and contents of the questionnaire for another researcher to be able to repeat the study in the future.

3 Do the results relate to the aims(s) and/or objective(s) of the study? Are the results robust and justified?

- ▸ There is an error in that the first line gives the total number of prisoners as 381 whereas the tables and other text describe 321 prisoners being invited to interview. This might indicate either a simple error in the report or an attempt to disguise the numbers of prisoners refusing to be interviewed.
- ▸ The table giving the SF36 results (Table 3) is very complicated and difficult to understand.
- ▸ There is no indication of what statistical test was used to calculate statistical significance and probabilities.
- ▸ Percentages rather than actual numbers of prisoners exercising were given so that it is impossible for the reader to check that the percentages have been calculated accurately.

4 Are there any biases in the design and execution of the study?

- ▸ There is no information about how the six prisons were selected nor how representative they were compared to others in the West Midlands or in the United Kingdom.

- ▸ The recruitment of prisoners by a mix of random selection and volunteers produced biased samples. The potential biases this created, if for example the volunteers were more health conscious, were not discussed anywhere in the paper.
- ▸ The prisoners' SF36 scores were compared with published norms for the general population. No account was taken of the likely different characteristics of prisoners with regard to previous level of education, literacy, occupational class, etc. and whether this might make comparison with average norms invalid.
- ▸ The method states that some prisoners were interviewed in a public room, throwing into doubt whether such interviewees would feel able to divulge sensitive information about themselves.
- ▸ There is no justification of why the SF36 was the scale chosen to measure general health of a prison population, nor whether it had ever been used for assessing prisoners before.
- ▸ Results for remand and convicted prisoners are mixed together with no indication of whether they are similar or why they are being combined.
- ▸ The 'chocolate gratuity' may have influenced prisoners in deciding to take part and in the answers they gave about their health.
- ▸ Comparison of prisoners' exercise habits with doctors and teachers does not make sense as they are such different populations.

5 Is the conclusion valid?

- ▸ No – the study has not proved that the general public are 'healthier' than prisoners. The results from prisoners in six prisons in one region in England cannot necessarily be extrapolated to the whole prison population of the United Kingdom. All the other types of potential biases to the results that are described above render such a conclusion invalid.

► The word 'healthier' has not been defined in the paper at all.

6 Are there any other concerns about the study?

► Information about chocolate rewards for completing the study is only admitted in the discussion and was omitted from the description of the method. Besides being wrongly placed, this raises suspicions about what else might have been omitted from the report.

► It is not clear why the researchers undertook such a study if they did not have officially approved access to prisoners' details.

So now critically appraise the report of a study you have identified from your search.

1 Are the aim(s) and/or objective(s) of the study clearly stated?

2 Is the design appropriate for fulfilling the aims – the population, the setting, the sampling technique, the type of study, the methods of measurement, avoidance of biases or confounding factors? Are all stages of the design described such that you could repeat the exact same study if you had a mind to do so?

3 Do the results relate to the aim(s) and/or objective(s) of the study? Are the results robust and justifiable? Can the results be generalised to your own circumstances? Are the results clear? Are there mistakes in the results?

4 Are there any biases in the design and execution of the study? Are they discussed in sufficient detail and are allowances made for their effects?

5 Are the conclusion(s) valid? What do they mean for your own practice?

6 Have you any other concerns about the study?

Critical appraisal of a qualitative research paper

Although qualitative research is not part of the hierarchy of evidence, it can provide a useful source of evidence. Qualitative research has been used extensively in the fields of nursing, professions allied to medicine (PAMs), mental health and the evaluation of the health service. Indeed, many nurses and PAMs searching for evidence in respect of their disciplines may find that while no quantitative research has been undertaken, there may be a number of published qualitative studies. Thus, it is essential that you are able to make a judgement about the quality of these types of studies as well. The following checklist and reminders about features you should consider is modified from Greenhalgh and Taylor (1997).[32]

1 Did the paper address an important clinical problem? Was the research question clearly formulated and defined?
There should be a clear statement about why the research was done and the research question that was addressed.

2 Is a qualitative approach the best method of answering this research question?
Qualitative research is useful for exploring beliefs, feelings and perceptions; for gaining a deeper understanding of an area; for exploring situations where little is known; for exploring sensitive issues; for gaining the 'whole picture'; and for allowing participants to speak for themselves. If this is what is being done, then a qualitative approach is almost certainly best. But think whether a quantitative approach, such as a randomised controlled trial (RCT) would have been more appropriate.

3 Is the setting/context for the research clear? How were the subjects selected? Is the sampling strategy described in detail? Is this strategy justified?
Qualitative research is about exploring the beliefs and gaining a deeper understanding of the experiences of a particular group of

people or individuals. The sample is therefore selected in order to include people from these groups. That is, people are chosen because they are part of that group, rather than being chosen at random or to represent the 'average' view.

4 Have the researcher's perspective, beliefs, experiences and background been taken into account?

'Researcher' or 'observer' bias is important in qualitative research as the interviewer's background, knowledge, experience, beliefs etc. may have an influence on the results of semi-structured interviews and focus groups. It is impossible to eliminate researcher bias, so the authors should address this problem by discussing the researcher's perspective and how this might have influenced the interpretation of the results.

5 What data collection methods were used and are these described in detail?

Rigorous reporting of methods in articles about qualitative research is particularly important, as each study is unique in design and analysis. The methods tell the 'story' that is needed to interpret the results. Hoddinott and Pill (1997)[33] suggest that you should ask the following questions:

▶ *are the researchers' roles and qualifications clear?*
▶ *are interviewer details given?*
▶ *is the paper explicit about how respondents were recruited, who recruited them and how the research was explained to them?*
▶ *is it explicit about whether the interviewer was known to the respondents and how they were introduced?*
▶ *is the interview setting clearly stated?*
▶ *were methodological issues about the influence of the interviewer on the data addressed?*

6 What methods were used to analyse the data? What quality control measures were implemented? Was an attempt made to test the validity of the results? Was an attempt made to test the reliability of the results?

There are various different methods of analysing qualitative data, e.g. content analysis and grounded theory. You should look for evidence that the researcher has analysed the data in a systematic way. Do the authors state that the data, e.g. transcripts, field notes or audio tapes, are available for independent review? The authors should have looked for cases which contradict the developing theories. The data should have been independently analysed by another researcher or a second researcher should have repeated the analysis.

7 Are the results credible? Are the findings clinically important?
Use your common sense and ask 'Do the results seem sensible and believable? Will they matter in practice?' You should also look at whether the authors present sufficient original data, e.g. verbatim quotes, and whether these are indexed to subjects so that they could be traced back and checked.

8 What conclusions were made? Are the conclusions justified by the results?
In qualitative research the results and the discussion are not separate as in quantitative research, as the results are an interpretation of the data. You can look for evidence that the conclusions are 'grounded in evidence', i.e. that they flow from the findings, how comprehensible the explanations are, how well the analysis explains why people behave in the way they do, and how well the explanation fits with what is already known.

9 Can the findings be transferred to other clinical settings?
Qualitative research is often criticised for only being applicable to the setting in which it was conducted. However, if true theoretical sampling rather than simply convenience sampling has been used, then the results are likely to be more transferable.

The checklist outlined above is not as all-encompassing or universally applicable as a checklist for critically appraising quantitative research, as qualitative research is 'by its very nature, non-standard, unconfined, and dependent on the subjective experience of both the researcher and the researched'.[32] This checklist sets some useful ground rules which may be enhanced by information given in other sources.[33-37]

Critically appraise a review

Now that you have learnt to critically appraise a research report, try your hand at appraising a review. Refer back to the explanations about randomised controlled trials, probability, confidence limits or other scientific terms described in the earlier text if necessary. The same rules apply for carrying out a survey of all research about a topic as for individual research papers. The specific question being addressed must be stated explicitly, the subject population (relevant research reports) identified and accessed, appropriate information obtained in an unbiased fashion (by using specific criteria to identify which research reports should, and should not, be included in the review) and the final conclusions should relate to the evidence obtained from the research reports included in the review related back to the primary survey question.

Look particularly for information in the review to reassure you of the following:

► The topic and purpose of the review are specified.
► The search methods used to find evidence relating to the question should be stated. The review of the literature should be comprehensive – reasonable efforts should have been made to identify and include relevant studies by consulting a range of databases and tracking down 'grey' material such as that in books, from conference proceedings, consensus statements or annual reports.
► The studies included in the review should be relevant and appropriate to the main subject or issue being addressed.
► Only similar data have been combined from different studies with similar subject characteristics, circumstances and methodologies. The methods used to combine the findings of the studies included in the review should be stated.
► There should be enough details about the subjects, populations, settings and other important factors for you to be able to decide whether the review's results and conclusions will be relevant to your particular circumstances.

▶ The criteria used to define whether or not a study was included in the overview should be stated clearly in the methods section. The researchers should have adhered to those explicit inclusion criteria, avoiding any bias in their method of selection.

▶ The results should be presented clearly in a scientific way. The results should be understandable, numbers in tables should add up, and it should be obvious how any analyses were derived.

▶ The authors should describe how the quality of the papers was assessed – how many people assessed each paper, whether they were blinded to other researchers' opinions, what criteria of quality were used, whether these criteria were valid, reliable and reproducible, and whether they adhered to the criteria.

▶ The results should be relevant to the declared aim of the review.

▶ The results should be generalisable – the significance of different biases should be considered and their implications discussed. The author(s) should give a critical analysis of the scientific rigour of the studies in the review, with all interpretative remarks being justified.

▶ The results should be comprehensive. Negative as well as positive findings in the different studies should be described. The range of confidence limits gives more information than a mere probability statistic.

▶ The conclusions should be based on an overview of the data and/or analyses of all the studies included in the review.

▶ The outcomes should indicate clearly any modifications that should be made to future healthcare practice based on the evidence presented in the review.

If you want to practise your critical appraisal skills obtain a copy of the following review:

▶ Waddell G, Feder G, Lewis M (1997) Systematic reviews of bed rest and advice to stay active for acute low back pain. *Br J Gen Pract.* **47**: 647–52.

Read through the article first to get a feel for it. Then read it again conscientiously absorbing the details and making notes as ideas and concerns come to mind. Now use the information given above, writing down your answers. The whole critical appraisal exercise should take you about three hours. Turn over and read how *we* reviewed this journal paper.

▼

It may be hard to convince your colleagues even when you've got the evidence.

Our review of Waddell G, Feder G and Lewis M (1997) Systematic reviews of bed rest and advice to stay active for acute low back pain. *Br J Gen Pract.* 47: 647–52

This published review was prepared for the national *Guidelines on Acute Low Back Pain*, an important and relevant problem in primary care. The following critique reflects the views of the authors and colleagues who attended the clinical effectiveness workshops. It is difficult to dissociate fact and interpretation in the critical appraisal of published papers and as several of the comments are matters of interpretation and opinion, you may well disagree with our critique.

Is the topic and purpose of the review clearly specified?

Yes. The aim was to review all randomised controlled trials of *bed rest* and of *advice to stay active* for acute back pain.

Were the search methods used comprehensive?

The search strategy was clearly stated and included searching Medline, Embase, hand searching and tracking down 'grey' materials. However, search of CINAHL was not included, which would have extended the search to include relevant literature from nursing and allied health disciplines, such as occupational therapy and physiotherapy.

Did the review address a clearly focused issue?

No. The inclusion criteria were too vague. For example, one of the inclusion criterion stipulated 'back pain of up to three months duration', but in some papers included in the review, the patients had had back pain for a few days, in others they had had pain for months. The inclusion criteria stated that trials of advice had to be set in 'primary care'. However, a very broad definition of primary care was used, e.g. three papers were set in occupational health clinics and emergency rooms.

The subjects in the bed rest studies and the advice populations were very different. That is, the settings, length of follow-up, different outcome measures (most of which were irrelevant according to Table 3), and on the whole, smaller samples were used in the *bed rest* papers compared to those about trials of *advice*.

Some papers concerned primary care, while others concerned hospital outpatient care. They included studies of patients with recurrent attacks, acute exacerbation of chronic back pain and sciatica. These are all groups of patients for whom optimum care may well be different and some may benefit from bed rest whilst other groups may not. They should have focused on a particular group or groups of patients, symptoms or settings.

There was no discussion of outcomes and the difficulties in measuring them. To sum up a paper as pain 'worse' or 'better' ignores the difficulties in assessing pain over a period of weeks. The most severe pain experienced or the duration of pain above a certain level, the average pain score, pain at rest or pain on activity are all important features.

Did the authors look for the appropriate papers to include in the review?

No. They should have been more focused. For example, they could have identified a clinical question such as 'Should patients with acute onset back pain be advised to rest in bed until the pain subsides, or should they be encouraged to stay active?' Then they should have searched for papers that reported trials comparing these two alternatives. Instead they treated *bed rest* and *advice* to stay active as separate interventions and carried out two separate reviews.

Although the authors noted the problems with two of the papers and discussed them separately, they still included them in their review. For example, the paper by Pal *et al.* (1986) compared bed rest and continuous traction with bed rest and sham traction, which is a trial of traction and not a trial of bed rest at all. These papers should have been excluded.

The authors state in the method that back schools were excluded, however one of the papers reviewed (Linequist *et al.*, 1984) is a trial of a back school.

Do you think the important, relevant papers were included?

No, papers on end-point evaluation have not been considered.

If the results of the review have been combined was it reasonable to do so?

No, the studies have too little in common.

Did the authors do enough to assess the quality of the included studies?

No. There were too many dubious features of the scoring method used. The weighting of the criteria used for methodological scoring seems to have been accepted uncritically by the authors since it had been used in two other systematic reviews of back pain management. For example, an intention-to-treat analysis is one of the items (N) included in the methodological scoring system in Table 2. This is an essential feature, as a study loses nearly all of its credibility if it lacks this, and not just 5 points out of 100 as in the scoring system used by Waddell *et al.* 'Placebo controlled' is another one of the items (J) in the methodological scoring system. However, it is difficult to see how trials of bed rest and advice to stay active can be scored as to whether they are placebo controlled and how placebo bed rest might be arranged. A further problem with the methodological scoring is that the total sum in Table 2 is 100, yet the weightings given only add up to 95.

There is no substantive reason why co-interventions such as appropriate analgesia should be avoided in a study of back pain. To be realistic a trial protocol should allow appropriate analgesia, but should endeavour to ensure that patients in both groups are managed using the same guidelines with respect to analgesia. Use of analgesia could be an appropriate end-point to study.

What is the overall result of the review?

It is unclear because of the numerous flaws. The diversity of the studies in this area suggests that a more traditional type of review might be better, where papers are grouped under headings.

How precise are the results?

They only give results as 'better' or 'worse'. More precision is needed.

There are also several major mistakes. There is an inconsistency between Tables 2 and 3 in the total sum possible for the methodological scoring item F, which is given as 12 in Table 2 and 17 in Table 3. This accounts for the total adding up to 95 and not 100 as stated.

In Table 4 the asterisks and crosses in the last two entries appear to be mixed up. The asterisks should be crosses and the crosses should not be there.

Under *Methodological Quality*, the Spearman's rank correlation coefficient of 0.72 should not be interpreted as showing the rankings were similar – a value of 0.9 would be required.

The reporting of the results seems biased. In Tables 4 and 5 there are several instances where results are given as 'NS' (not significant) and several where the NS is elaborated on as 'slower recovery NS'. Where there is elaboration on NS, the detail, for example 'slower recovery (NS)', favours the final conclusion of the review. There must have been information available about all the 'NS' results and so the authors seem to have been selective in how much detail they present in order to favour their final conclusions.

Can the results be applied and generalised?

No, there are too many flaws. Furthermore, many of the studies included were not in primary care.

Were all important outcomes considered?

No, there is too little detail about outcomes, such as pain. Few of the important outcomes, such as time off work, were considered in the bed rest arm of the review.

Are the benefits worth the harms and costs?

This is unclear, given the flaws outlined above.

Apply the evidence

You have identified your problem, posed your question with help from colleagues at work, searched for the best available evidence, judged the quality of the evidence, weighed the relative importance of any conflicting results, applied the evidence theoretically to your own circumstances and situation, and now you should be ready to apply the evidence in practice.

Clinicians have expressed concern about the dangers of adhering blindly to evidence in practice, and fears that evidence-based practice might be regarded as the be-all and end-all as far as decisions about the cost-effective delivery of health services go. Clinical judgement and common sense must be paramount in keeping evidence in perspective. The information forming the 'evidence' may be irrelevant, incomplete or inaccurate, or the 'evidence' may simply not be applicable in the particular clinical circumstances in question. The NHS has a long way to go in accumulating a bank of good and reliable information about current clinical care and best practices.

Sir Douglas Black[39] warned about giving undue primacy to the evidence generated in randomised controlled trials. They may provide the best sort of evidence for evaluating the benefits of alternative medications, but they are not necessarily the best way of identifying evidence for resolving more complex human health issues.

Evidence-based management has an even weaker information base than evidence-based clinical practice. It must be right to encourage practice managers and other health service managers to adopt a research culture with a questioning approach. This will encourage them to reflect about what is happening, how and why, and to compare management practices.

So bear all this in mind as you think about applying the evidence you have gained from your search to your particular clinical situation. You may like to think of making changes from the perspective of an individual clinician, a practice or unit, or a primary care group (PCG) or trust.

Diary of your progress in searching for evidence

Complete this summary of progress to date and your action plan for how you propose to introduce any changes in your working practices.

Write a summary of:

1 your problem (be as specific as possible so that you can measure the outcomes of any changes against this baseline position):

2 your question:

3 your search method – where you searched (databases, people):

4 the types of your best evidence (systematic review, randomised controlled trials, controlled trials, reports, conference proceedings, expert opinions):

5 give three titles of the most relevant and appropriate publications or sources that you found:

6 your conclusion(s) from the best evidence available in answer to your question:

7 the change(s) that you propose to make yourself or that others should make, as a result of the evidence you have obtained and the conclusion(s) you have drawn:

Action plan

People to whom you have fed back the results of the evidence:

Have you already written a timetabled action plan?   *Yes / No*

The baseline position:

Whom have you involved in discussions about the change(s) you propose?

Change(s) proposed:

People whom the proposed change(s) will affect:

Additional resources that will be required (people, premises, time, money, skills, etc.):

The timetable is:

Who will do what:

Advantages or health gains expected:

Disadvantages or losses (opportunistic costs) that may happen:

How and when the changed situation will be monitored again:

Barriers to change

Once evidence has been gathered, projects have been completed and necessary changes discussed there can still be many barriers to overcome before worthwhile changes can happen.

The King's Fund PACE[6] initiative has identified the following barriers to change:

▶ others' lack of perception of the relevance of your proposed change (you should have realised this during your initial consultations with colleagues before you began)
▶ lack of resources to implement the change (time, staff, skills, equipment)
▶ short-term outlook of work colleagues
▶ conflicting priorities – without additional resources, changes have the potential to cause work overload or opportunity costs
▶ difficulties in measuring outcomes – it is difficult to find acceptable worthwhile health outcomes that are easily measured
▶ lack of necessary skills (forward planning is needed)
▶ no tradition of multidisciplinary working (this problem can probably only be surmounted with a culture change)
▶ limitations of research evidence on effectiveness (there's a lot more research about problems than there is about effective solutions)
▶ perverse incentives (a common flaw in the way the NHS functions)
▶ the intensity of others' contribution that is required (again consult early, get everyone on board and encourage everyone to 'own' your project).

And so …

▶ anticipate the strength of evidence you will need to convince your colleagues that the efforts and costs of change will be worthwhile – to them and the patients. Do this through clinical governance – understand how to make clinical governance work for you in the next chapter.

Read more about the lessons to be learnt in how to make successful changes happen.[6]

What clinical governance means and how to put it into practice

Clinical governance is inclusive, making quality everyone's business, whether they are a doctor or a nurse, manager or member of the administrative staff, a patient or a strategic planner. We need to know where we are now and where we want to get to if we are to drive up standards of healthcare. Clinical effectiveness and clinical audit are central to this process.

Clinical governance 'is doing anything and everything required to maximise quality'.[40] It is about finding ways to 'implement care that works in an environment in which clinical effectiveness can flourish by establishing a facilitatory culture' where at the same time, underperformance is weeded out.[41–43]

Components of clinical governance

The components of clinical governance are not new. Bringing them together under the banner of clinical governance and introducing more explicit accountability for performance is a new style of working. The reception given to clinical governance has ranged from an enthusiastic welcome to the cautious warning that innovations that improve quality may increase rather than decrease costs. Carefully evaluating your work and demonstrating subsequent improvements in patient care, will enable you to form your own view about the place of clinical governance.

The following 14 themes are core components of professional and service development which taken together form a comprehensive approach to providing high-quality healthcare services and clinical governance. These are illustrated in the tree diagram:[43]

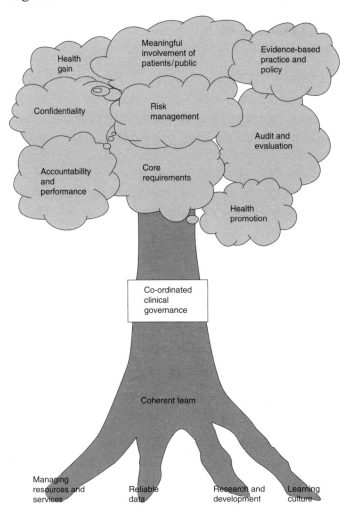

Figure 1   'Routes' and branches of clinical governance (© 2000 Chambers and Wakley)

If you interweave these into your individual and workplace-based personal and professional development plans, you will have addressed the requirements for clinical governance at the same time.[43]

1 **Learning culture**: in the practice, the primary care organisation, the trust and the NHS at large.
2 **Research and development culture**: throughout the health service.
3 **Reliable and accurate data**: in the practice, the primary care organisation and the NHS as a seamless whole.
4 **Well managed resources and services**: as individuals, as a practice, as a primary care organisation or trust, across the NHS and in conjunction with social care and local authorities.
5 **Coherent team**: well integrated teams within a practice, across a practice, in the primary care organisation or trust.
6 **Meaningful involvement of patients and the public**: in a practice or the NHS as a whole, including users, carers and the general population.
7 **Health gains**: activities to improve the health of patients in a practice, between practices, in the primary care organisation or trust, and different geographical areas of the NHS.
8 **Confidentiality**: of information in consultations, in medical notes, between practitioners.
9 **Evidence-based practice and policy**: applying it in practice, in the primary care organisation or trust, in the district, across the NHS.
10 **Accountability and performance**: for standards, performance of individuals, the practice, primary care organisation or trust, health authority/board and the NHS, to the public and those in authority.
11 **Core requirements**: good fit with skill mix and whether individuals are competent to do their jobs, communication, workforce numbers, morale at practice level, across the NHS.

12 **Health promotion**: for patients, the public, opportunistic and in general, targeting those with most needs.
13 **Audit and evaluation**: for instance, of changes, of individuals' and practices' performance, of the primary care organisation's or trust's achievements, of district services.
14 **Risk management**: pro-active review, follow-up, risk management, risk reduction.

The challenges to delivering clinical governance

Delivering high-quality healthcare with guaranteed minimum standards of care for users at all times, is a major challenge. At present the quality of healthcare is patchy and variable. We aren't very good at detecting underperformance, and then taking the initiative and rectifying it at an early stage. The small number of clinicians who do underperform exert a disproportionately large effect on the public's confidence. Causes of underperformance in an individual might relate to a lack of knowledge or skills, poor attitudes or ill health. A lack of management capability is nearly always an important contributory factor to inadequate clinical services or the provision of healthcare.

We need to understand why variation exists and explore ways of reducing inequalities. Variation in the quality of healthcare provided is common – between different practices in the same locality, between staff of the same discipline working in the same practice or unit, between care given to some groups of the population rather than others. There may be up to four-fold differences in rates of referral to hospital for a particular condition, between one doctor and another for example; some practices have attached social workers and community psychiatric nurses whilst others do not, for instance.

Good practice means understanding and managing risk – both clinical and organisational aspects. Identifying new cases of important conditions such as diabetes and undertaking audit more systematically will reduce the risks of omission – in detection and clinical management. The common areas of risk in providing healthcare services are thought to be:[44]

▶ out of date clinical practice
▶ lack of continuity of care
▶ poor communication
▶ mistakes in patient care
▶ patient complaints
▶ financial risk – insufficient resources
▶ reputation
▶ staff morale.

Clinical governance offers a co-ordinated approach to overcoming these areas of risk through the blend of clinical and organisational improvements to the quality of healthcare practice.

We need to agree on indicators of performance that are acceptable to clinicians and managers alike. It is often said that we tend to use outcomes that are the easiest to measure but which mean least in terms of the real quality of patient care.

Enhancing your personal and professional development

Education and training programmes should be relevant to service needs, whether at organisational or individual levels. Continuing professional development (CPD) programmes need to meet both the learning needs of individual health professionals and the wider service development needs of the NHS. You should no longer opt for CPD activities according to what you *want* to do, but rather, what you *need* to do. Clinical governance underpins professional and service development.[41]

Lifelong learning and CPD are integral to the concept of clinical governance and that includes everyone in a practice working towards agreed learning goals that are relevant to service development.

> **individual personal development plans**
> will feed into a
> **workplace or practice-based personal and
> professional development plan**
> that will feed into
> **the organisation's business plan**
> all
> **underpinned by clinical governance**[45]

Good morale and job satisfaction are prerequisites of learning and effective working, and should be nurtured by targeted personal and professional development plans. Clinical governance should be creating a culture and working environment where people thrive and feel fulfilled by their work.

The Royal College of General Practitioners has developed a variety of awards that recognise the high standards of quality of care achieved by a practitioner or a practice team – Membership and Fellowship by Assessment, Quality Practice Award, Quality Team Development and others. These require sustained CPD coupled with demonstrable high standards of care – clinical governance principles are integral to the process. The principles that underlie the Quality Team Development process are:[46]

- the criteria for assessment reflect the needs of patients
- professional self-regulation is the most effective and acceptable method of maintaining good professional practice
- the ethos should be educational, developmental and supportive
- every member of the primary healthcare team can take part
- the focus is the team, its functioning and the services it provides
- assessment should be multidisciplinary
- there should be local ownership and delivery.

1 How evidence-based care, clinical effectiveness and other components of clinical governance fit together: the practitioner's, the practice's or the unit's perspective[43]

Learning culture

You cannot learn about the cultural changes needed for providing multidisciplinary, team-based healthcare in the modern health service by sitting passively in a lecture. You need to experience the learning and interact with others who will be part of that new culture. Historically, health professionals have been keener to attend lectures than interactive educational activities such as organised small group sessions or informal teaching in their workplaces.

> The type or mode of education and training should be relevant to the topic of the learning and the characteristics or circumstances of the 'students'.

Maximising learning about the new requirements of the NHS will involve:

▶ setting up in-house formal and informal education and training opportunities

▶ everyone creating personal development plans that incorporate all modes of learning: reading and reflecting, shadowing others, small group discussions, online materials, as well as lectures and seminars

▶ a practice or directorate wide approach to a topic so that a portfolio of experience is built up to which everyone contributes – useful for revalidation and re-registration of team members' professional qualifications.

Applying research and development in practice

One of the most common research and development activities undertaken by health professionals is a questionnaire survey of their patients. A poorly designed patient satisfaction survey will give you meaningless results so that all the time and effort spent on the satisfaction survey is wasted, and changes made as a result of such a survey still do not satisfy the patient population. Patient satisfaction questionnaires are commonly used in hospital and general practice, as a hybrid of research and audit. Novices may mistakenly believe that undertaking a questionnaire survey is one of the simplest and easiest methods.

> Using a questionnaire is full of pitfalls and it is one of the most difficult techniques for gaining a true or valid answer to the question posed.

To try and ensure that a patient satisfaction survey is a meaningful exercise:

▶ use a questionnaire that has been tried and tested by someone else and is valid for a general practice setting
▶ make sure that the questions are relevant and appropriate to the purpose of the enquiry
▶ use questions which have an easily answered format with simple choices of response
▶ use appropriate language likely to be understood by all respondents, with translations into other languages if there are non-English speakers in your target population
▶ avoid leading questions that imply you are expecting a particular answer, otherwise respondents will tend to give the answer implied as being the 'right' one because they want to please you
▶ pilot your draft questionnaire to detect problems with your questions or method.

Reliable and accurate data

Clinicians, patients and administrators need reliable and accurate data to connect individuals or their healthcare records to other knowledge that is relevant to the care of the patient.
Set standards for a general practice:

► keep records in chronological order
► summarise medical records; within specified time period for records of new patients
► review dates for checks on medication; with audit in place to monitor standards adhered to and plan for underperformance if necessary
► establish chronic disease registers and keep them updated
► use computers for diagnostic recording
► record information from external sources – hospital, other organisations – relevant to individual patients or the practice as a whole.

Well managed resources and services

The things you need to achieve best practice should be in the right place at the right time and working correctly everytime.
Set standards in your workplace for:

► access to premises and availability of services for people with special needs such as those with sensory and visual impairment
► provision of routine and urgent appointments
► access to and provision for referral for investigation or treatment
► pro-active monitoring of chronic illness and disability
► alternatives to face-to-face consultations
► consultation length.

The six primary care services to which the public requires access are: information, advice, triage and treatment, continuity of care, personal care and other services.[47] Minimising inequalities and the outcomes of new skill mix models are two prime concerns at the heart of considerations about access and evaluating standards, especially with respect to:

► level of access versus quality of care received
► access for those who demand more versus equity of access for all based on need
► an impersonal service versus continuity of care versus personal care
► a demand-led (by patients) service versus a service that is prioritised or rationed
► access to one particular member of the care team, first or above others.

Systems should be designed to prevent and detect errors. So keep systems simple and sensible, and inform everyone how systems operate so that they are less likely to bypass the system or make errors.

Coherent team work

Teams do produce better patient care than single practitioners operating in a fragmented way. Effective teams make the most of the different contributions of individual clinical disciplines in delivering patient care. The characteristics of effective teams are:

► shared ownership of a common purpose
► clear goals for the contributions each discipline makes
► open communication between team members
► opportunities offered for team members to enhance their skills.

A team approach helps different team members adopt an evidence-based approach to patient care, by having to justify their approach to the rest of the team.[48]

The experiences of teamwork on the Wirral[48]

The team was composed by a family support worker employed by the voluntary sector joining a community psychiatric nurses team. They found that the factors that helped the team to work well were:

▶ that each member of the team had a separate function
▶ joint training which cemented the team, but obstacles from different employer arrangements had to be overcome
▶ interdisciplinary differences of opinion about patient care being welcomed as a way of increasing debate and generating a wider range of options for care.

Meaningful involvement of patients and the public

The terms 'user' and 'public' are employed here to include patients or users, carers, non-users of services, the local community, a particular sub-group of the population and the general public.

If user involvement and public participation is done well it should result in:

▶ reductions in health inequalities
▶ better outcomes of individual care
▶ better health for the population
▶ better quality and more locally responsive services
▶ greater ownership of health services
▶ a better understanding of why and how local services need to be changed and developed.

Public participation may be organised at five levels and you should aim for true participation at the fifth level whenever possible:[49]

▶ **Level 1**: information exchange
▶ **Level 2**: consultation: the public and patients express their views but the consultant makes the decisions

▶ **Level 3**: support: the public decides what to do and others support them in doing it
▶ **Level 4**: deciding together: thinking and planning together
▶ **Level 5**: acting together: putting plans into action together.

A meaningful public consultation involves the exchange of information between the healthcare providers and the general public, obtaining a representative opinion as a result that feeds into the local decision-making process of healthcare services or whoever is sponsoring the consultation.

How to go about undertaking meaningful consultation[50]

Be clear about:

▶ the purpose of the exercise: is it important and is it necessary?
▶ the type and identity of the population to whom the purpose relates
▶ how to reach and engage the target population
▶ the extent and mode of information exchange required prior to consultation
▶ the implications of the methods you employ in the consultation – what outputs you expect from the consultation
▶ how you will act on the results of the consultation
▶ how you will feedback the outcome of the consultation exercise
▶ how you will evaluate the consultation exercise.

You may have to trade-off a relatively cheaper method of consultation that engages with fewer people or with a less representative section of the population sub-group; if you do, you will need to understand what biases are arising and make allowances for those biases when you interpret the results of the consultation.

Health gains

Taking the example of coronary heart disease (CHD).

Modifiable risk factors for CHD include: cigarette smoking, raised blood pressure, body composition, lack of physical exercise, total serum cholesterol and excessive alcohol consumption.

Maximising the reduction in patients' risk factors for CHD in general practice, for example, will involve:

► identifying patients who will benefit from medical interventions, e.g. you might identify patients for secondary prevention of ischaemic heart disease by extracting information from repeat prescriptions for nitrates and/or aspirin, looking through medical records for patients with specific conditions (e.g. post- myocardial infarction, angina) or who have been classified as having CHD and entered on the practice computer

► targeting those patients once identified in systematic ways and auditing the results of your campaign

► discussing CHD risks as a practice team so that everyone has a similar understanding of the risks and benefits, gives out consistent messages and recommends similar interventions

► using the most up-to-date interventions with best outcomes, e.g. in your approach to smoking cessation

► remembering that a patient's perceived risk or susceptibility is an important determinant of whether the patient takes preventive action.

Confidentiality

Confidentiality is a component of clinical governance that was often overlooked in the workshops which informed this book. Experienced health professionals and managers may assume that junior or new staff know all about confidentiality and, of course, they may not. There are many tricky situations where one person asks for information about another's medical condition – test results or a progress report – where it is not clear cut as to whether this information should be supplied or withheld, or even if the person asked should acknowledge that the person enquired about is under their care. If the person in question is terminally ill and within a few days of death, the health professional will want to prepare the relatives; if the person with the terminal illness is functioning well, then their medical attendants will not be able to share medical information without the patient's express permission.

The Caldicott committee report[51] describes principles of good practice to safeguard confidentiality when information is being used for non-clinical purposes:

► justify the purpose
► do not use patient identifiable information unless it is absolutely necessary
► use the minimum necessary patient identifiable information
► access to patient identifiable information should be on a strict need-to-know basis
► everyone with access to patient identifiable information should be aware of his or her responsibilities.

Evidence-based culture: policy and practice

The key features of whether or not local guidelines worked in one initiative were that:[52]

► there was multidisciplinary involvement in drawing them up
► a well described systematic review of the literature underpinned the guidelines with graded recommendations for best practice linked to the evidence
► ownership was nurtured at a national and local level
► a local implementation plan ensured that all the practicalities (time, staff, education and training, resources) were foreseen and met, stakeholders were supported, predictors of sustainability addressed – guideline usability, individualising guidelines to practitioners and patients.

Clinicians may rebel against new policies that they perceive as being out of line with patients' needs, and policy makers may become frustrated at the intransigence of those in practice – if there is a gulf between those driving policy and those responsible for practice. The evidence base justifying health policy and management decisions in relation to a particular service is just as important as the evidence base for the clinical care component of the service or the education of staff providing that service.

> Incorporating research-based evidence into everyday practice should promote policies on effective working and improve quality and a clinical governance culture.

- Be sure of the evidence for a proposed policy and the best way to implement it. Search for the evidence or set up a formal evaluation where there is insufficient evidence of the best way.
- Consult widely and early when any policy decision is being made, demonstrating how the input to that consultation was incorporated into the final policy.
- Base management and policy decisions on accurate information.
- Negotiate necessary changes in the organisation and management of practice and carefully cascade information about the changes throughout the practice team or organisation.
- Provide adequate resources to underpin strategies to change practice, such as people to promote that change who have the right levels of knowledge and skills.
- Incorporate monitoring and evaluation of the change from the planning stage and throughout the activity.
- Find ways to maintain and reinforce the new practices, e.g. reminder systems, educational outreach programmes.
- Disseminate information about the change in ways that are appropriate to the nature and setting of the participants.

Accountability and performance

Health professionals do not always realise that they are accountable to others from outside their own professions, particularly GPs with their self-employed status. But in fact they are accountable to:

- the general public – who are entitled to expect high standards of healthcare
- the profession – to maintain standards of knowledge and skills of the profession as a whole
- the government and employers – who expect high standards of healthcare from the workforce.

> Health professionals who believe that they are not accountable to others may be reluctant to collect the evidence to demonstrate that they are fit to practise, and that their working environment is fit to practise from, the basis of the evidence for revalidation of their professional qualifications. In addition, they may not co-operate with central NHS requirements such as the National Service Frameworks.

Identify and rectify underperformance at an early stage by:

- regular appraisals (at least annually) linked into clinical governance and personal development plans. Appraisal is a process of regular meetings between manager and staff member with support for the benefit of the member of staff
- detecting those who have significant health problems and referring them for help
- systematic audit that detects individuals' performance as opposed to the overall performance of the practice team
- an open learning culture where team members are discouraged from covering up colleagues' inadequacies so that problems can be resolved at an early stage.

> Many misunderstandings arise between patients and doctors that have potential or actual adverse consequences. Fourteen categories of misunderstanding were identified in one study of prescribing relating to patient information unknown to the doctor, doctor information unknown to the patient, conflicting information, disagreement about attribution of side effects, failure of communication and relationship factors. This study demonstrated how dependent clinical management is on good organisational systems manned by non-clinical staff, and how important it is that patients participate in the consultation.[53]

Health promotion

People may under-estimate relative risks as applied to themselves and their own behaviour, e.g. many smokers accept the relationship between smoking tobacco and disease, but do not believe that they are personally at risk. People usually have a reasonable idea of the *relative risks* of various activities and behaviours, although their personal estimates of the *magnitude* of risks tend to be biased – small probabilities are often over-estimated and high probabilities are often under-estimated.[54]

> You need to understand the terms used to be able to extrapolate the messages from a research paper to explain the risks and benefits to others. You need critical appraisal skills to be able to form an opinion as to whether you can depend on the results from a research study.

Audit and evaluation

We should be looking for ways of assessing qualities like kindness, empathy, clinical reasoning, listening skills, as well as more tangible measures of the quality of care.

Clinicians may see the performance assessment framework as a management tool that is not particularly relevant to their clinical practice; this attitude will obstruct a coherent improvement programme if managers and clinicians have different goals.

> The NHS performance assessment framework has six components which include: health improvement, fair access, efficiency, effective delivery of appropriate care, user/carer experience and health outcomes.[55]

▶ Communicate the meaning and implications of the performance assessment framework and indicators of achievement to individual practices and practitioners.
▶ Incorporate the components of the framework into district or primary care group/trust wide audits of practice performance, feeding back comparable data to individual practices.

Analysis of critical incidents should focus on organisational factors as well as the performance of particular individuals.

Core requirements

You cannot deliver clinical governance without well trained and competent staff, the right skill mix of staff, a safe and comfortable working environment, all providing cost-effective care.

Following published referral guidelines may increase healthcare costs, which should be justifiable as cost-effective care when all direct and indirect costs are taken into account.

Your healthcare team can do much under the umbrella of clinical governance to respond to the national challenges to improve:

▶ partnership: working together across the NHS to ensure the best possible care

- performance: acting to review and deliver higher standards of healthcare
- the professions and wider workforce: breaking down barriers between different disciplines
- patient care: access, convenient services, empowerment to take a full part in decision making about their own medical care and in planning and providing health services in general
- prevention: promoting healthy living across all sections of society and tackling variations in care.

Risk management

Risk management in general practice or a trust mainly centres on 'facts' rather than 'values' or 'preferences'. These are the facts about what the probability is that a hazard will give rise to harm – how bad is the risk, how likely is the risk, when will the risk happen if ever and how certain are we of our estimates about the risks. This applies just as much whether the risk is an environmental or organisational risk in the practice, or a clinical risk.[54]

Communicating and managing risks with individual patients is very much about finding ways to explain risks and elicit people's values and preferences, so that all these dimensions can be incorporated into the decisions they make themselves, to take risks or choose between alternatives that involve different risks and benefits.[54] A well functioning system through which patients can make complaints and receive feedback on the outcome should allow the practice or unit to reduce the risk of a recurrence.

Take travel health, for instance, as an example of risk management which requires consideration of clinical and organisational risks, that are minimised or eliminated.

> *The risks* of acquiring infections from travelling abroad are greater if people are not aware of the specific risks of disease and do not take appropriate precautions.

Risk management to reduce the chances of a traveller contracting an avoidable disease from abroad involves:

► having a consistent policy in your practice team for advice given for types of vaccination for specific countries and situations

► being able to signpost patients to travel advice centres and sources of information for further help, e.g. yellow fever centre

► encouraging patients to complete their courses of immunisation after they have returned from holiday to give them longer lasting immunity

► good stock control of immunisations stored in the surgery, so you do not have an excessive quantity that then exceeds its 'best before' date and you do not run out of stocks and disappoint patients.

> Chemoprophylaxis to avoid malaria is only one part of a preventive approach – awareness of the risk by traveller and doctor, reducing bites from mosquitoes and awareness of the residual risk with prompt diagnosis and treatment of clinical malaria are all components of risk management.

2 How evidence-based care, clinical effectiveness and other components of clinical governance fit together: the primary care group or trust perspective[43]

The 14 components of clinical governance described apply just as much to the approach required by a PCG or PCT in the same way as for practices and individual health professionals. But they must also set up:

► clear lines of responsibility and accountability for the overall quality of clinical care in their constituency

▶ a systematic approach to monitoring and developing clinical standards in practices
▶ a comprehensive programme of quality improvement systems including workforce planning and development
▶ education and training plans
▶ clear policies aimed at managing risk
▶ integrated procedures for all professional groups to identify and remedy poor performance
▶ a culture where education, research and sharing good practice are valued.[56]

Clinical governance will be part of a culture of learning and the organisation will have an ethos of participation – for staff and patients to engage in quality improvement.

The action plan that follows was the result of one clinical governance sub-committee of a West Midlands PCG, brainstorming their position at an awayday held in summer 2000. When they took stock of the baseline assessment of the achievements and omissions of the 22 practices in their constituency, they realised that they needed to do a great deal to invest in and build up an infrastructure, and to educate and support staff, before they could expect to establish a culture of clinical governance where the working environment facilitated best practice. Their reflections and plans may apply equally well to a PCT or other NHS trust.

Action plan for the next 12 months for XXXX Primary Care Group – an example from the West Midlands

i Establish and organise clinical governance infrastructure:

► support practice clinical governance leads: cascade of leads in all practices and other organisations in the constituency

► organise the gathering of reliable data: efficient input and retrieval of data, prioritising data

► provide protected time in practice for: building up infrastructure, undertaking quality improvement and support

► keep PCG's requirements of practices simple in short term: aim for co-operation rather than verification of their performance, for now

► help practices understand what is required of them

► demonstrate benefits of clinical governance, e.g. by compiling an example portfolio of evidence for revalidation of professional qualifications, disseminating real examples of good chronic disease management and better patient management

► infrastructure in practices will be individualised according to practice characteristics.

ii Suggest clinical topics as example areas to build clinical governance infrastructure at practice (or unit) level, e.g. management of coronary heart disease (CHD):

► practice profile template: staffing, premises, facilities at the practice, recent audit activity, level of patient involvement and participation, special services offered or planned, professional development activities, how

continued opposite

information technology is used, risk management approach

▶ clinical checklist of best practice: checklist around CHD theme will include standards and timetabled programmes for health promotion, lifestyle, FH, smoking, medication, and standards for access for routine, semi-urgent, emergency consultations (i.e. a mix of proactive/reactive standards)

▶ gain consensus across the PCG about what standards are acceptable

▶ establish baseline of what professionals currently do, to highlight gaps and duplication in relation to standards

▶ get feedback from patients about current services (via published literature and local consultation exercises)

▶ identify what works from the Cochrane database

▶ summarise existing standards and protocols, looking at how they match with 'gold' standards given in the Cochrane database

▶ identify the skill base of staff across the PCG's constituency in relation to CHD

▶ identify the core standards expected in primary care (for instance in the National Service Framework for CHD, the health improvement programme)

▶ feed back the above to practices and ask them to identify their timed action plans to deliver clinical and infrastructure goals, what resources/support they need (include checklist of what they could ask for) and who leads in the practice on that clinical topic, education and training, clinical governance and other priority areas.

iii Areas in which the PCG could offer practical support:

▶ staff training

▶ help to set up disease registers and other common information systems

continued overleaf

- shared use of specialist nurses
- IT training to set up recall systems, sharing expertise between highly developed practices and needy ones
- raising awareness about the meaning and implementation of clinical governance
- initial prioritisation of most needy practices from baseline assessment of performance
- disseminate information to practices – written material, seminars, workshops, personal contact etc
- scope of skill base within PCG – expertise of staff and good models of practice
- run educational sessions linking with PCG tutors and multidisciplinary training. Trawl what is available and where there are gaps commission education – local workshops; link to scheduled training (receptionist, nurse training); arrange training about practice-based learning plans; training about skills in user involvement/ public consultation; link to roadshows for patients and the public
- identify practice needs against defined standards, i.e. against agreed practice checklists of good practice considering infrastructure, clinical management of CHD
- patients' and public's views actively sought at PCG level and disseminated to practices
- introduce innovations by demonstrating their significant benefits, based on evidence.

iv Evaluate activities: agree short-term and longer-term outcomes; aim to reach surrogative targets as per agreed standards; measure achievement of improved care/ services against standards.

The threats to a coherent clinical governance programme that the clinical governance sub-committee perceived were:

► lack of practice consensus and teamwork
► lack of understanding of priorities
► 'What's the point' if no resources for change?
► 'blame' culture – way of thinking
► geographic isolation of some staff and practices
► lack of trust and information about skills between health professions
► suspicion of small practices that they will be criticised or have their priorities swamped by larger practices
► fear of new things/deficit in skills to cope with rapid change
► lack of time to fit new things in and get involved
► practices may find providing comparative data threatening
► clinical governance sub-group may be seen as 'know it alls' and 'do it alls' by other local practices who then leave them to it
► few practitioners have personal development plans and many are unsure how best to proceed to blend clinical governance in with continuing professional development
► there is a lack of ownership of the importance of clinical governance by 'ordinary' practitioners
► clinical governance is seen as a threat and as a top down imposition by some practices (not all)
► lack of multidisciplinary culture or ownership – not all members of the practice team see themselves with a part to play in clinical governance
► there are anxieties about how information on performance will be used and interpreted
► staff sickness levels may create variations in the delivery of services and blips of underperformance
► lack of systematic staff training
► the many initiatives may raise patient expectations above the capacity to deliver
► staff turnover in some practices may be detrimental, e.g. loss of experience in using disease registers and recall systems

- some small isolated practices may find it hard to share information and resources with peers
- lack of opportunities/willingness to learn about clinical governance in some practices
- low level of public involvement, so standards are set by healthcare staff rather than the public
- practices not all using the same IT hardware or recording systems
- lack of co-ordination and updating of data about morbidity, consultations etc
- worries about identifying weaknesses as source of blame
- health professionals may not see the wider context of the contributions of non-health organisations to improving health, nor understand each others' roles or the potential of the services each offers.

One review of how clinical governance was evolving in NHS trusts concluded that clinical governance could be simplified into five themes:[57]

1 policy emphasis on national consistency
2 accountability being at the heart of clinical governance
3 co-ordinating and linking audit, clinical effectiveness, complaints and risk management with an over-arching and coherent system of quality improvement and assurance
4 the assumption of responsibility for the management of poor performance and the promotion of clinical quality by chief executives leading to appraisal systems within trusts, external inspection, hospital doctors taking part in national audit
5 collaboration and teamwork between professionals.

One hospital approach to clinical governance was to reform the senior committee structure to reflect:[58]

▶ leadership at different levels
▶ multidisciplinary style
▶ active co-ordination of the different elements of the committee, and of the hospital
▶ sharing of work across the service.

To achieve this, lead roles and responsibilities were allotted so that:

▶ evidence-based practice was led by a consultant psychiatrist
▶ risk management was led by a forensic psychologist
▶ a nurse manager led on policy and procedure
▶ the senior occupational therapist led on clinical audit
▶ a general manager led on user issues and complaints.

3 How evidence-based care, clinical effectiveness and other components of clinical governance fit together: a district wide perspective[43]

The district perspective is to take an overview, to check that national priorities are being satisfactorily translated into local prioritised action and that the anticipated outcomes of clinical governance are happening to reduce inequalities, and raise standards of healthcare in a uniform way across the district. The district perspective will be centred around the health improvement programme which should have been put together and actioned by all the NHS family and relevant non-health organisations.

Publishing information about achievements as league tables of professionals or organisations may worry patients and the public unnecessarily; and annoy health professionals who feel that any disadvantages about the context in which they work have not been fully taken into account. Highlighting any aspect of clinical governance may alarm the public in any case, if they think that any new initiative indicates that there are currently a lack of quality standards in place.

Clinical governance is a compulsory feature of all publicly funded healthcare services but not of the private sector. This may cause tensions between the two if staff drain from one sector to another in response to different working conditions or financial incentives.

Clinical governance should be integral to any district strategies that promote high-quality healthcare. The strategy should encourage equity between primary care organisations and between trusts in the same district and a co-ordinated approach to quality improvement between the NHS and other organisations with an influence on health – education, local authority departments such as housing and police, voluntary organisations etc.

The following example of one district's primary healthcare strategy highlights many of the principles of clinical governance. A yearly implementation plan encourages the acute and community trusts, the community health council, the council for voluntary services, social services and others from outside the NHS to work with the chief executives of the PCGs/PCTs to agree responsibility for specific parts of the annual programme. This programme ties in with the primary care investment plan and other priorities, and is underpinned by clinical governance.

Implementing a district wide healthcare strategy[59]

The vision for healthcare in North Staffordshire is one where high-quality primary healthcare services:

- are centred on the needs of the person, the family and the community
- promote health and self-care of individuals and the community
- improve access and reduce inequalities in health and healthcare in the locality
- improve and maintain the health and social circumstances of individuals

underpinned by investing in quality, partnerships, education, communication by:

- listening to and involving the public, users and carers in providing and planning services
- adequate numbers of well educated and trained, motivated staff
- working in partnership with other agencies
- integrated care, basing interventions on evidence/best practice
- making the best use of resources
- establishing good communications at all levels
- being flexible to allow for new ways of working to meet new challenges
- working from good quality premises with disabled access and facilities
- integrating health promotion in primary healthcare for individuals and the community
- empowering individuals and organisations.

Once you've tried to apply clinical effectiveness – you'll want to do it again!

► EVALUATE YOUR NEWLY GAINED KNOWLEDGE AND SKILLS IN CLINICAL EFFECTIVENESS AND CLINICAL GOVERNANCE

Evaluate how much you have learned by doing this programme and compare your answers to questions 1 and 2 below with the equivalent questions in your initial self-assessment of your knowledge and skills about the topic at the beginning of this book.

Please circle as many answers as apply or fill in the information requested.

1 How confident do you feel *now* that you know enough about clinical effectiveness to be able to:

Ask a relevant question?	*Very*	*Somewhat*	*Not at all*
Undertake a search of the literature?	*Very*	*Somewhat*	*Not at all*
Find readily available evidence?	*Very*	*Somewhat*	*Not at all*
Weigh up available evidence?	*Very*	*Somewhat*	*Not at all*
Decide if changes in practice are warranted?	*Very*	*Somewhat*	*Not at all*
Make changes in practice as appropriate?	*Very*	*Somewhat*	*Not at all*

2 Which databases(s) have you used in this programme?

Medline   Cochrane   Internet   Other (what?)

3 What level of evidence did you find in answer to your question (or main question if you posed more than one question)?

Strong evidence from at least one systematic review of multiple, well-designed randomised controlled trials (RCTs).

Strong evidence from at least one properly designed RCT of appropriate size.

Evidence from well-designed trials without randomisation.

Evidence from well-designed non-experimental studies from more than one centre or research group.

Opinions of well-respected authorities, based on clinical evidence, descriptive studies or reports of expert committees.

No evidence at all.

4 To whom have you given a report about the evidence you found?

Colleagues at work   Friends/family   Bosses (managers) or GP at work   Other (who?)

5 What is/are the outcome(s) of you asking your main question and finding the evidence?

Made change(s) to an aspect of work – if so, please describe what change(s) you have made or plan to make, who was involved in deciding to make the change(s), who is involved in the new change(s), whether you need any more resources or training, and how you will review the change(s):

Decided against making any change(s) to any aspect of work – if so, why did you decide not to make any change(s) and who was involved in that decision?

Other outcome – what?

6 How will you use your new-found knowledge about clinical effectiveness in the future?

7 A practice nurse and therapist with whom you work have been given the task of triaging patients requesting emergency appointments. The nurse sees all the patients except for those complaining of musculoskeletal pain of some sort, who are referred to the physio at the next appointment. Lots of patients are complaining to you how difficult it is to see a doctor nowadays, and the nurse and therapist moan because too little time has been allocated to see these extra patients and the additional training they've been promised has not materialised. What do you do? (Circle all that apply.)

Nothing – it's not your responsibility.

Inform the patients how to complain.

Log the patients' complaints and report them to the practice manager.

Encourage the nurse and therapist to take their concerns to the next practice team meeting.

Support the nurse and therapist in reviewing the operation of the new system with the practice manager and clinical governance lead.

(Hopefully, your own response will reflect the position that everyone working in the NHS is responsible for the quality of care their team provides.)

8 You have just been appointed as the clinical governance lead in your workplace. What are your roles and responsibilities likely to be and how will you go about promoting a positive culture of clinical governance among your team members?

   Write down your answers – you can glean the information you need from Stage 6 which is the chapter on applying clinical governance in practice.

► USEFUL PUBLICATIONS OF EVIDENCE ALREADY AVAILABLE

Some evidence is already available, so it is not necessary to appraise all the evidence yourself. The following resources will be useful.

Bandolier is a UK newsletter published by the NHS Executive, Anglia and Oxford, which provides key evidence about the effectiveness of healthcare and keeps purchasers up-to-date with both local and national initiatives. It is free within the NHS in England and Wales. It is available in full text on the Internet at http://www.jr2.ox.ac.uk/Bandolier/. Non-NHS subscriptions are available from Hayward Medical Communications, Rosemary House, Lawades Park, Kentford, Newmarket, Suffolk, CB8 7PW. To register, email bandolier@pru.ox.ac.uk.

Clinical Evidence is a compendium of evidence on the effects of common clinical interventions, published by the BMJ Publishing Group. It is updated and expanded every six months and summarises the best available evidence about the prevention and treatment of a wide range of clinical conditions. Plus points are that its contents are driven by questions rather than by the availability of research evidence and so it identifies gaps in the evidence, leaving you to make your own decisions. Annual subscription costs £75 for individuals. However, an electronic prototype of Issue 1, June 1999 is free on the Internet. For more details see http://www.evidence.org/index-welcome.htm.

Clinical Guidelines from the US Agency for Health Care Policy. Full text guidelines and summaries of the systematic reviews on which they are based. See http://text.nlm.nih.gov.

Drug & Therapeutics Bulletin provides independent evaluations of drugs and other medical treatments and management issues. It is available from the Consumers' Association, Castlemead, Gascoyne Way, Hertfordshire SG14 1LH or at http://www.which.net.

Effective Healthcare Bulletin provides summaries of systematic reviews produced by the NHS Centre for Reviews and Dissemination and is designed to help NHS decision makers make more informed decisions by presenting the latest available information on the effectiveness of particular health service interventions. The bulletins are based on a systematic review and synthesis of the literature on clinical effectiveness, cost effectiveness and acceptability of health service interventions. It is available from the Subscriptions Department, Pearson Professional, PO Box 77, Fourth Avenue, Harlow CM19 5BQ or at the CRD website http://www.york.ac.uk/inst/crd.

Effectiveness Matters is produced by the NHS Centre for Reviews and Dissemination to complement *Effective Health-Care. Effectiveness Matters* provides updates on the effectiveness of important health interventions for practitioners and decision makers in the NHS. It covers topics in a shorter and more journalistic style, summarising the results of high quality systematic reviews. Topics have relevance to primary healthcare. It is distributed free within the NHS – to subscribe inform the Publications Office. The full text of most of the *Effectiveness Matters* series can be viewed on the Internet at http://www.york.ac.uk/inst/crd or are available from the NHS Centre for Reviews and Dissemination, University of York, York YO1 5DD.

Evidence-Based Medicine provides critical appraisals of systematic reviews and primary research, with a commentary from a clinical expert. The journal is available on the *Best Evidence* database at http://hiru.hirunet.mcmaster.ca/acpjc and from the BMJ Publishing Group, PO Box 299, London WC1H 9TD.

Guide to Clinical Preventative Services (2e). Evidence-based recommendations on preventive services. It is available at http://text.nlm.nih.gov/.

Journal of Clinical Effectiveness publishes papers on clinical effectiveness, evidence-based practice, guidelines and audit. Contact details: Financial Times Professional Ltd, PO Box 77, Subscriptions (Journals) Department, Harlow, Essex CM19 5BQ. Tel: 0800 801405.

MeReC Bulletin provides reviews of new drugs aimed at GPs covering issues of safety, effectiveness, cost, appropriateness and acceptability. It is available from the Medicines Resource Centre, Hamilton House, 24 Pall Mall, Liverpool L3 6AL.

Netting the Evidence is part of the Cochrane Library that advises on where to find information on the Internet on using evidence in practice. See http://www.shef.ac.uk/~scharr/ir/netting.html.

NHS Economic Evaluation Database provides critiques of published economic evaluations. It is available from the NHS Centre for Reviews and Dissemination, University of York, York YO1 5DD or on the Internet at http://nhscrd.york.ac.uk/welcome.html.

Organisations

Aggressive Research Intelligence Facility (ARIF)
ARIF is a specialist unit funded by the NHS Executive, West Midlands. The role of the unit is to improve the incorporation

of research findings into population level healthcare decisions in the NHS by helping healthcare workers access and interpret research evidence, particularly systematic reviews of research. Although ARIF has a regional role, it will attempt to help all callers. The website provides summaries of the research information ARIF has uncovered in response to requests received. The website is at: http://www.hsrc.org.uk/links/arif/.

National Institute for Clinical Excellence (NICE)

NICE provides NHS patients, health professionals and the public in England and Wales with authoritative, robust and reliable guidance on current 'best practice'. This is regularly updated and offers guidance on appraisals of new and existing health technologies, the clinical management of specific conditions and clinical audit. Information about the Institute and its work is available on their website at: www.nice.org.uk.

NHS Centre for Reviews and Dissemination (CRD)

CRD is a sibling organisation of the UK Cochrane Centre, funded by the Department of Health to provide information on the effectiveness and cost-effectiveness of treatments and the delivery and organisation of healthcare. CRD carries out systematic reviews, provides a database of good quality reviews, offers a dissemination and information service and helps to promote research-based practice in the NHS. CRD plays an important role in disseminating the contents of Cochrane reviews to NHS decision makers. It provides an information and enquiry service on reviews and economic evaluations for healthcare professionals, purchasers and providers, NHS managers, information providers, health service researchers and consumer organisations. Its main outputs are: *Effective Healthcare Bulletins*; *Effectiveness Matters*; Database of Abstracts of Reviews of Effectiveness (DARE); NHS Economic Evaluation Database (NHS EED); and the Health Technology Assessment (HTA) Database. NHS Centre for Reviews and Dissemination, University of York, York YO1 5DD. Tel: 01904 433707. Email: revdis@york.ac.uk. The website is at: http://www.york.ac.uk/inst/crd/.

Useful websites include:

▸ CASP (Critical Appraisal Skills Programme):
http://www.public-health.org.uk/casp/
▸ Centre for Evidence-Based Medicine:
http://cebm.jr2.ox.ac.uk/
▸ Clinical Governance Research and Development Unit:
http://www.le.ac.uk/cgrdu
▸ Cochrane Collaboration Home Page:
http://hiru.mcmaster.ca/cochrane/default.htm
▸ EBM Informatics Home Page:
http://hiru.hirunet.mcmaster.ca/ebm/
▸ EBM toolbox at:
http://cebm.jr2.ox.ac.uk/
▸ IDEA Topics List:
www.ohsu.edu/bicc-informatics/ebm/ebm_topics.htm
▸ Netting the Evidence:
http://www.shef.ac.uk/~scharr/ir/netting.html
▸ 'NEW' TRIP database:
http://www.ceres.uwcm.ac.uk/frameset.cfm?section=trip
▸ Trawling the net:
http://www.shef.ac.uk~scharr/ir/trawling.html
▸ Ukpractice.net Ltd: http://www.ukpractice.net

There is also a very good email discussion group: evidence-based-health@mailbase.ac.uk.

To join send the following email to mailbase@mailbase.ac.uk. Leave the subject field empty and type the message 'join evidence-based-health Jo Bloggs'. To get the list of discussions send the email. Website at http://www.mailbase.ac.uk.

Further reading

Baker M, Maskrey N and Kirk S (1997) *Clinical Effectiveness and Primary Care*. Radcliffe Medical Press, Oxford.

Chambers R and Wakley G (2000) *Making Clinical Governance Work for You*. Radcliffe Medical Press, Oxford.

Crombie I (1996) *The Pocket Guide to Critical Appraisal*. BMJ Publishing Group, London.

Greenhalgh T (1997) *How to Read a Paper: the basics of evidence-based medicine*. BMJ Publishing Group, London.

Jones R and Kinmonth AL (eds) (1995) *Critical Reading for Primary Care*. Oxford University Press, Oxford.

The King's Fund (1998) *Turning Evidence into Everyday Practice*. The King's Fund, London.

Kobelt G (1996) *Health Economics: an introduction to economic evaluation*. Office of Health Economics, London.

Lilley R (1999) *Making Sense of Clinical Governance*. Radcliffe Medical Press, Oxford.

Muir Gray JA (1997) *Evidence-Based Healthcare*. Churchill Livingstone, Edinburgh.

Ridsdale L (1995) *Evidence-Based General Practice*. Saunders, London.

Sackett D, Richardson S, Rosenberg W and Haynes RB (1997) *Evidence-Based Medicine*. Churchill Livingstone, Edinburgh.

van Zwanenberg T and Harrison J (eds) (2000) *Clinical Governance in Primary Care*. Radcliffe Medical Press, Oxford.

Wilson T (ed) (1999) *The PCG Development Guide*. Radcliffe Medical Press, Oxford.

Computer language

Internet acronyms:

AFAIK: as far as I know
AKA: also known as
BTW: by the way
FAQ: frequently asked question
FYI: for your information
IM(H)O: in my (humble) opinion
NRN: no response necessary
TIA: thanks in advance
TTFN: ta ta for now
WRT: with respect to.

► REFERENCES

1 NHS Executive (1996) *Promoting Clinical Effectiveness.* NHS Executive, London.

2 Hicks N (1997) Evidence-based health care. *Bandolier.* **4**(5): 8.

3 Sackett DL, Rosenberg WM, Gray J, Haynes RB and Richardson WS (1996) Evidence-based medicine: what it is and what it isn't. *BMJ.* **312**: 71–2.

4 Haynes B, Sackett D, Gray JM, Cook D and Guyatt G (1996) Transferring evidence from research into practice: 1. The role of clinical care research evidence in clinical decisions. *Evidence-Based Medicine.* **November/December**: 196–7.

5 Haynes B, Sackett D, Gray JM, Cook D and Guyatt G (1997) Transferring evidence from research into practice: 4. Overcoming barriers to application. *Evidence-Based Medicine.* **May/June**: 68–9.

6 The King's Fund (1997) *Turning Evidence into Everyday Practice.* The King's Fund, London.

7 McColl A, Smith H, White P and Field J (1998) General practitioners' perceptions of the route to evidence-based medicine: a questionnaire survey. *BMJ.* **316**: 361–5.

8 Samuel O (1997) Evidence-based general practice: what is needed right now. *Audit Trends.* **5**: 111–15.

9 Prescott K, Lloyd M, Douglas HR *et al.* (1997) Promoting clinically effective practice: general practitioners' awareness of sources of evidence. *Fam Pract.* **14**: 320–3.

10 Paterson C (1997) Problem setting and problem solving: the role of evidence-based medicine. *J Roy Soc Med.* **90**: 304–6.

11 le Vann T (1998) Are we doing any good? *Monitor.* **4 February**: 19.

12 Kernick D (1997) Why GPs should be wary of evidence-based medicine. *Pulse.* **13 December**: 48–50.

13 Houghton G and Mendes da Costa B (1997) *EBM: a multidisciplinary educational needs assessment in the West Midlands* (unpublished). This is an internal paper intended for local circulation only. It is available from the Evidence-supported Medicine Union, 27 Highfield Road, Edgbaston, Birmingham B15 3DP.

14 NHS Executive West Midlands (1995) *GRIP Kit, 1995.* The GRIP Group, NHS Executive West Midlands.

15 Aggressive Research Intelligence Facility (ARIF) (1997) *General Information Leaflet.* The University of Birmingham, 27 Highfield Road, Edgbaston, Birmingham B15 3DP. http://www.hsrc.org.uk/links/arif/.

16 Royal College of General Practitioners (1993) *Portfolio-based Learning in General Practice: a report of a working group on higher professional education.* Occasional Paper 63. RCGP, London.

17 Treasure W (1996) Portfolio-based learning pilot scheme for general practitioner principals in South East Scotland. *Education for General Practice.* 7: 249–54.

18 Burrows P and Millard L (1996) Personal learning in general practice. *Education for General Practice.* 7: 300–5.

19 Millman A, Lee N and Kealy K (1995) The Internet. ABC of Medical Computing series. *BMJ.* **311**: 440–3.

20 *The Cochrane Library.* Update Software Ltd, Summertown Pavilion, Middle Way, Summertown, Oxford OX2 7LG. http://www.cochrane.co.uk.

21 Brenner SH and McKinnin EJ (1989) CINAHL and Medline: a comparison of indexing practices. *Bulletin of the Medical Library Association.* 77: 366–71.

22 Okuma E (1994) Selecting CD-ROM databases for nursing students: a comparison of Medline and the Cumulative Index to

Nursing and Allied Health Literature (CINAHL). *Bulletin of the Medical Library Association.* **82**: 25–9.

23 Watson MM and Perrin R (1994) A comparison of CINAHL and Medline CD-ROM in four allied health areas. *Bulletin of the Medical Library Association.* **82**: 214–16.

24 Kiley R (1997) Medical databases on the Internet – part 2. *J Roy Soc Med.* **90**: 679–80.

25 Kiley R How to get medical information from the Internet. *J Roy Soc Med.* **90**: 488–9.

26 Kiley R (1998) Evidence-based medicine on the Internet. *J Roy Soc Med.* **91**: 74–5.

27 *Oxford Clinical Mentor* is available from Janet Caldwell, Oxford University Press, Great Clarendon Street, Oxford OX2 6DP.

28 Muir Gray JA (1997) *Evidence-Based Healthcare.* Churchill Livingstone, Edinburgh.

29 Kobelt G (1996) *Health Economics: an introduction to economic evaluation.* Office of Health Economics, London.

30 Rowlands J, Morrow T, Lee N and Millman A (1995) Online searching. ABC of Medical Computing series. *BMJ.* **311**: 500–4.

31 Greenhalgh T (1997) The Medline database. How to Read a Paper series. *BMJ.* **315**: 180–3.

32 Greenhalgh T and Taylor R (1997) How to read a paper: papers that go beyond numbers (qualitative research). *BMJ.* **315**: 740–3.

33 Hoddinott P and Pill R (1997) A review of recently published qualitative research in general practice. More methodological questions than answers? *Family Practice.* **14**(4): 313–19.

34 Blaxter M (1996) Criteria for evaluation of qualitative research. *Medical Sociology News.* **22**: 68–71.

35 Mays N and Pope C (eds) (1996) *Qualitative Research in Health Care.* BMJ Publishing Group, London.

36 Mays N and Pope C (2000) Qualitative research in health care. Assessing quality in qualitative research. *BMJ.* **320**: 50–2.

37 Murphy E, Dingwall R, Greatbatch D, Parker S and Watson P (1998) Qualitative research methods in health technology assessment: a review of the literature. *Health Technology Assessment.* **2**.

38 Waddell G, McIntosh A, Hutchinson A, Feder G and Lewis M (1999) *Low Back Pain Evidence Review.* Royal College of General Practitioners, London.

39 Black D (1998) The limitations of evidence. *Journal of Royal College of Physicians of London.* **32**: 23–6.

40 Lilley R (1999) *Making Sense of Clinical Governance.* Radcliffe Medical Press, Oxford.

41 Department of Health (1997) *The New NHS: modern, dependable.* The Stationery Office, London.

42 Department of Health (1998) *A First Class Service: quality in the new NHS.* Health Services Circular HSC (98)113. Department of Health, London.

43 Chambers R and Wakley G (2000) *Making Clinical Governance Work for You.* Radcliffe Medical Press, Oxford.

44 Lilley R and Lambden P (2000) *Making Sense of Risk Management.* Radcliffe Medical Press, Oxford.

45 Wakley G, Chambers R and Field S (2000) *Continuing Professional Development in Primary Care: making it happen.* Radcliffe Medical Press, Oxford.

46 Royal College of General Practitioners (2000) *Quality Team Development.* RCGP, London.

47 Royal College of General Practitioners (2000) *Access to General Practice Based Primary Care.* RCGP, London.

48 Dunning M, Abi-Aad G, Gilbert D *et al.* (1999) *Experience, Evidence and Everyday Practice.* King's Fund, London.

49 Taylor M (1995) *Unleashing the Potential: bringing residents to the centre of regeneration.* Joseph Rowntree Foundation, York.

50 Chambers R (2000) *Involving Patients and the Public: how to do it better.* Radcliffe Medical Press, Oxford.

51 Department of Health (1997) *Report of the review of patient-identifiable information.* In: *The Caldicott Committee Report.* Department of Health, London.

52 Donald P (2000) Promoting local ownership of guidelines. *Guidelines in Practice.* **3**: 17.

53 Britten N, Stevenson F, Barry C *et al.* (2000) Misunderstandings in prescribing decisions in general practice: qualitative study. *BMJ.* **320**: 484–8.

54 Mohanna K and Chambers R (2001) *Risk Matters in Healthcare: communicating, explaining and managing risk.* Radcliffe Medical Press, Oxford.

55 NHS Executive (1999) *The NHS Performance Assessment Framework.* Department of Health, London.

56 NHS Executive (1999) *Primary Care Trusts: establishing better services.* NHSE, London.

57 Dewar S (1999) *Clinical Governance Under Construction.* King's Fund, London.

58 James A (2000) Making space for clinical governance. *Impact in Bandolier.* **7**(3): 5–6.

59 North Staffordshire Health Authority (1998) *Primary Health Care Strategy.* North Staffordshire Health Authority, Stoke-on-Trent.

▶ INDEX